Praise for
*Into the Mouths*

"*Into the Mouths of Babes* is a fabulous book full of absolutely everything needed to provide babies with the nutritional foundation to set the stage for a lifetime of health and well-being."

~ Christiane Northrup, MD
Ob/Gyn physician and author of the *New York Times* bestsellers:
*Women's Bodies, Women's Wisdom* and *The Wisdom of Menopause*

"Susan Tate's *Into the Mouths of Babes* sets the highest standard for books on how to nourish our little ones. Her work is comprehensive, heartfelt, informative, and easy to read and implement. Susan elegantly weaves together all the practical details that parents need to know to feed a child in the best possible way: kitchen set-up, recipes, shopping, nutritional insights, food allergies, and much more. But this book will provide you with more than just great nutrition strategies. It teaches parents how to raise a child who's healthy in body, mind, heart, and soul. Every mom deserves a copy of this wonderful book, and every newborn deserves to benefit from the wisdom that Susan Tate has to share. Highly recommended!"

~ Marc David, Nutritional Psychologist
Founder of the Institute for the Psychology of Eating
and best-selling author of *Nourishing Wisdom* and *The Slow Down Diet*

"Whether one adopts the entire approach or merely uses some of the ideas herein, this book is a prime resource for parents who need to tailor their children's diets away from the high load of sugared, salted, processed, chemically laden, high-animal-protein-containing foods to the wiser food choices spelled out here. Healthy food for kids need not be sterile, flat, and no fun. Susan Tate has seen to it that tasty *and* healthy foods can be primary staples, a vital ingredient for optimal nourishment."

~ Ray C. Wunderlich, Jr., MD, PhD
Preventive Medicine Specialist

"As a health coach and mother of two, I come from a nutrition and health-centered background and feel I have a steady grasp on what it means to feed my children healthy foods. AND I feel reinvigorated and refocused by the information and inspiration Susan offers in every page and recipe. Her book is brimming with practical tips for feeding your children—from breastfeeding to introducing solids to making your own yogurt—and steeped in spiritual principles, what she calls the Seven Sacred Nutrients. Susan emphasizes self-care as a key to ensuring our children develop healthy views on food and body image, stating, 'Providing your child with the best nourishment possible may mean it's not always about the food.' Reading this book is like having a loving godmother in your kitchen, holding your hand while you learn to deeply enjoy feeding your family, encouraging and uplifting you as a mother or father set with the daunting task of raising a healthy person into the world. Her non-judgmental and holistic approach to healthy cooking empowers parents to embrace this adventure, with a food mill in one hand and a spice jar filled with Love in the other. Thank you, Susan, from the bottom of my Mama Bear heart."

~ Kate Short Lindsay
Holistic Health Coach and Mother of Two


*"Into the Mouth of Babes* is a joy to read. Susan shares her wisdom as a mom, health educator, and passionate participant of life. Her thought-provoking yet readable and accessible style is evident throughout the book. As a mother, whole foods dietitian, wellness educator and coach, I welcome this resource to share with the families I work with and those preparing for parenting. Busy parents can use it to find quick and easy recipes, wisdom and perspective on a long day, or to find out more about specific topics of interest such as starting solids or breastfeeding."

~ Wendy Vigdor-Hess, RD, RMT, WellCoach
Author of *Sweetness Without Sugar: A Resource Guide for Delicious Dairy-,
Egg-, and Gluten-Free Treats Made with Healthy Sweeteners*


"I wish this book had been available when my son was an infant! Not only did I crave the nutrition wisdom Susan offers in this book, I really could have used her comforting words of support and encouragement for self-care. This book needs to be in the hands of every mother. Period."

~ Deborah Kern, PhD
Health Scientist and author of *Everyday Wellness for Women*
and co-author of *Create the Body Your Soul Desires*

"With obesity and type 2 diabetes on the rise in children, this book is so important. What a wonderful support tool for new parents to nourish their children well."

~ Dr. Karen Wolfe, MBBS (Sydney), MA
Author of *Is Your Lifestyle Killing You? The 8 Simple Steps for Lasting Weight Loss and Optimal Health* and co-author of *Create the Body Your Soul Desires*

*"Into the Mouths of Babes* is a practical, nourishing guide to raising your baby on natural foods. I am in LOVE with the book! Susan Tate shares her wisdom, as a mother and as a health educator, to bring a foundation of wellness into your home that will benefit your children for a lifetime."

~ Kathryn Simmons Flynn
Author of *Cooking for Fertility* and Founder of Fertile Foods

"As a mother, this book was an invaluable asset to me when I was feeding my own baby. As a birth doula, I feel strongly about empowering families by providing them with thorough, balanced, and accurate information about their pregnancy, birth, and parenting choices. I am genuinely thrilled to recommend this book for anyone who works with new families or who has young children of their own to nourish."

~ Priya Curtis
Mother, Birth Doula

"As a first time mother-to-be and nutritional novice, I feel well prepared to feed my baby having read *Into the Mouths of Babes*. Susan Tate's philosophy of serving whole foods mixed with 'sacred nutrients' like Love and Respect empowers me to tap my inner wisdom for guidance on what to eat and *how* to eat. I now daydream of mindful, joyful mealtimes with my new family. The recipes in this book are simple, healthful, and sound fun! Banana Crunchsicles, anyone? Best of all, Susan prepares us to feed more than babes, offering us rules of thumb and recipes to help our babies' transition to healthy toddlers, children, and teens. This book will be on the kitchen counter for life!

~ Gretchen Musgrove
Expectant Mother

"*Into the Mouths of Babes* has been my 'bible' for feeding my baby, and I'm proud to say I have never bought baby food! Thanks to Susan Tate, I've had a practical, easy-to-follow, fun, and inspiring guide to introducing my baby to a lifetime of healthy eating."

~ Sarah Thomssen Brixey
Founder of LiveLong Wellnesss

"Quite simply, Susan Tate is brilliant! She has written the book my soul was longing for when I had an infant. Love beams from every page as she so eloquently combines the science of nutrition and the essence of a joy-filled life. It so clearly captures the beauty of healthy nourishment and self-care! How on earth she has put together such a beautiful book with content that is so simple to understand *and* doable is amazing to me. This will be the book I gift to all the families I work with as a holistic birth doula."

~ Donette Morris
Mother, Yoga Therapist, and Holistic Birth Doula

"I love, love, love the contents of this book. It is written with such love, care and knowledge of the needs of babies, caregivers, families, and human kind. There are subtleties that I would not have understood just a year ago, but now I fully appreciate. And I know over time, this will be a resource I can go back to and get more nuggets of good information."

~ Nani Courten
Kunmi's Mum

"There are some inventive ideas for 'toddle food' . . . as well as recipes for children who are allergic to eggs, milk, or wheat. The author writes in an appealing, chatty style." (From a review of the first edition.)

~ *Publishers Weekly*

# INTO THE
# MOUTHS OF BABES

REVISED AND UPDATED

# INTO THE MOUTHS OF BABES

## A whole foods nutrition guide to feeding your infants and toddlers

## SUSAN TATE

*Into the Mouths of Babes is a fabulous book—full of absolutely everything needed to provide babies with the nutritional foundation to set the stage for a lifetime of health and well-being.*

Christiane Northrup, MD
Author of *Women's Bodies, Women's Wisdom* and *The Wisdom of Menopause*

BALBOA.
PRESS
A DIVISION OF HAY HOUSE

Balboa Press books may be ordered through booksellers or by contacting:
Balboa Press
A Division of Hay House
1663 Liberty Drive
Bloomington, IN 47403
www.balboapress.com
1-(877) 407-4847

Because of the dynamic nature of the Internet, any web addresses or links contained in this book may have changed since publication and may no longer be valid. The views expressed in this work are solely those of the author and do not necessarily reflect the views of the publisher, and the publisher hereby disclaims any responsibility for them.

Edited by Lee Revere
Cover design and chapter illustration by Crista Goddard, © 2013
Author photo by Donna Lowe

The author of this book does not dispense medical advice or prescribe the use of any technique as a form of treatment for physical, emotional, or medical problems without the advice of a physician, either directly or indirectly. The intent of the author is only to offer information of a general nature to help you in your quest for emotional and spiritual well-being. In the event you use any of the information in this book for yourself, which is your constitutional right, the author and the publisher assume no responsibility for your actions.

Any people depicted in stock imagery provided by Thinkstock are models, and such images are being used for illustrative purposes only.
Certain stock imagery © Thinkstock.

ISBN: 978-1-4525-7334-2 (sc)
ISBN: 978-1-4525-7336-6 (hc)
ISBN: 978-1-4525-7335-9 (e)

Library of Congress Control Number: 2013907691
Library of Congress Cataloging-in-Publication Data
Tate, Susan Into the Mouths of Babes/Susan Tate.—3rd ed.
p. cm.
Includes bibliographical references.
1. Infants-Nutrition 2. Vegetarian children 3. Baby foods.
1. Title

Printed in the United States of America.

Balboa Press rev. date: 06/20/2013

## Also by Susan Tate

*Wellness Wisdom: 31 Ways to Nourish Your Mind, Body, & Spirit*

*AIDS & HIV Education: Effective Teaching Strategies**

*Working Together to Prevent Sexual Assault**
(with Mark S. Benn, PsyD)

*Written under her former name, Susan Tate Firkaly

# Table of Contents

For my children, grandchildren, and all the children of the world.

May all children be fed

May all children be healed

May all children be happy

May all children be loved

May all children be sheltered

May all children be educated

May all children be free

# In Gratitude

It is with an abundance of gratitude that I acknowledge those who contributed to the creation of this book.

**Prayers and blessings flow to . . .**

Helen and Ray Tate, my late parents, for the gift of life. You set the example of how to nourish and love in a most sacred and profound way.

Dr. Ray C. Wunderlich, Jr., who without hesitation so willingly agreed to write another highly complimentary foreword to welcome readers to this third edition.

Dr. Christiane Northrup, Marc David, Dr. Deborah Kern, Dr. Karen Wolfe, Kathryn Simmons Flynn, Kate Short Lindsay, Wendy Vigdor-Hess, Priya Curtis, Gretchen Musgrove, Sarah Thomssen Brixey, Donette Morris, and Nani Courten for creating time to read this manuscript and for providing such thoughtfully expressed and outrageously supportive endorsements.

Crista Goddard, for your talented graphic design skills in our co-creation of the book cover design. Thank you for how your heart flowed through your pen as you created the gentle pea vine illustration that added the perfect artistic touch to this edition.

Lee Revere, for your expert copyediting skills and invaluable insights on this manuscript. Your support, especially during the final week of manuscript preparation, saved me from throwing the computer out the window.

Ms. Lowe, thank you, Donna, for taking one more author photo of me. The sparkle in your eyes and the impishness behind the camera brings out the best in me.

My Team Northrup colleagues, whose vision of a healthier world inspires and supports the wellness of people across the globe. You shine.

My Nia students and the worldwide Nia community, for being such a powerful inspiration as I dance (and write) through life. And a special splash of gratitude to Debbie Rosas, co-creator of The Nia Technique, for permission to adapt her beautiful writing of "The Voice of Pleasure" into the words that flowed through me to craft "The Voice of Self-Care."

The many friends and family members who provided their constant love and support all through the years as each of these three editions emerged into print. I would need a separate book to list all of your names. If you are smiling when you read this, know you are included in this list.

My grandchildren, Abu and Aurora—the next generation of wise souls. What a kick it is to have you contribute recipes to this edition! Thank you for your wit, laughter, and love . . . and thank you to the mother of these precious ones, Peggy Farley, for your wondrous and expansive mothering heart.

My former husband, Michael Firkaly; thank you for all the love, for our children, for the laughter in the kitchen, and for your support during the writing of the earlier editions. In many ways, I couldn't have done this without you.

Nalani, for loving my son, for being all you are, and for being in my life.

Patrick, the amazing Austrian man who makes my daughter laugh and reflects the presence of nourishing love in her daily life.

Zack Orion and Molly Firkaly, the most spectacular children I could have ever wished for—oh, what you two have taught me! Thank you for the gift of watching you grow and flourish as the creative, compassionate, delightfully humorous, and wise individuals you are. You nourish me. You fill me up. I am so blessed to be your mother.

The Divine Nourisher of All, thank you, God, for my amazing life, family, and friends, and for the opportunity to share this wisdom to support the sacred nourishment of Your precious children.

# Foreword

Refreshing but especially reassuring is the news that Susan Tate's adult children consistently choose to eat healthy foods. Now, close to thirty years after her first edition of this book, the fact that her children have not become junk-food addicts is evidence that her loving, nutritional counsel supplies the needs of children without obsessive deviations that lack "staying power."

For health reasons, the latest guidelines for Americans advocate an increased consumption of vegetables, fruits, and whole grains. One could not find a better way to implement that wisdom than to start *today* with good feeding of the babes, toddlers, preschoolers, schoolers, and future parents. Hence the supreme value of this carefully detailed and documented book.

Some readers of this book may not elect to eat in an entirely vegetarian way. Nevertheless, the value of a high-quality diet as detailed herein cannot be overemphasized. Whether one aims to be vegan, lacto-vegetarian, lacto-ovo-vegetarian, or "near-vegetarian," the basic suggestions in Susan Tate's book are grist for the mill of good health. Her unique contribution is the combination of the best of academic learning with the experience of gentle caring for little people and the knowledge that "healthier eating" makes a difference.

In today's rapid-fire, often hectic society, one must honestly ask this question: "How many parents are actually going to bother to put aside established convenience-eating to make their children's meals when already prepared foods offer such an 'attractive' option?" The answer is that a growing wave (more than one-third of patients who see doctors) of health conscious individuals has already turned to so-called "alternative" medicine to manage their departures from health. Many more seek healthy choices to prevent illness and thus avoid the need for expensive, after-the-fact, high-tech diagnosis and treatment. At a time when such modalities as antioxidants, herbs, homeopathic remedies, massage, exercise, and prayer are increasingly used to blunt the accumulated ravages of stressful, fast-paced, convenience lifestyles, Susan Tate's counsel offers the practical dietary know-how that every family needs. Moreover, the marketplace today has responded so that healthy eating need not be the chore it once was.

Whether one adopts the entire approach or merely uses some of the ideas herein, this book is a prime resource for parents who need to tailor their children's diets away from the high load of sugared, salted, processed, chemically laden, high-animal-protein-containing foods to the wiser food choices spelled out here.

Healthy food for kids need not be sterile, flat, and no fun. Susan Tate has seen to it that tasty *and* healthy foods can be primary staples, a vital ingredient for optimal nourishment. My experience of over forty-five years of medical and pediatric practice strongly indicates that eating in this way can only result in fewer allergies, behavior disorders, infectious diseases, and later degenerative illness in those who—like Susan's children— continue the favorable eating habits that this book so cogently asserts.

The breadth and depth of Susan Tate's insights in this new edition of her book target the issues that must be addressed in building health. Her Seven Sacred Nutrients strike at the heart of the diseasing process, for, indeed, our offspring must grow with a diet of Joy, Wisdom, Respect, Quality, Safety, Pleasure, and Love, as well as with a broad variety of healthy foods.

Sherry Rogers, MD (*Total Wellness Newsletter*, November 2006) reminds us that the Columbia College of Physicians and Surgeons (my alma mater) has shown that over 95% of all diseases have two fundamental causes: diet and environment. *Into the Mouths of Babes* provides parents with the positive, shaping aspects of proper feeding, and its additional Seven Sacred Nutrients encourage a healthful surround. With diet and environment so addressed, how can our society fail to disseminate this text for all expectant mothers and their babies?

Ray C. Wunderlich, Jr., MD, PhD
St. Petersburg, Florida

# Preface to the Third Edition

When my daughter, Molly, encouraged me to update *Into the Mouths of Babes*, she provided the spark to light the way for this nourishing venture. "My friends are starting their families and I want them to have this information, Mama!" To have my daughter offer this inspiration and encouragement is a gift I cannot ignore. It didn't take me long to affirm, "Yes, this third edition is ready to be birthed." I'm thrilled to have thoroughly updated this book to share a gift of nourishment for you and your children.

Molly and her brother Zack provided the motivation for the original version close to thirty years ago. And now this mother is a grandmother. My days in the kitchen squirting my own breast milk into rice cereal are long gone. (Yes, I really did that!) However, you will still find me in the kitchen, joyfully creating nutritious foods to share with family and friends.

Somewhere around the middle of my first pregnancy, it occurred to me that I would have the task of deciding what to feed our baby. This was in 1976 and the information on how to feed a vegetarian baby was limited. While studying everything I could on pregnancy and childbirth through the eyes of a mother and a health educator, I began the search for answers to my many questions.

As my knowledge of infant nutrition expanded and scraps of paper overflowed my recipe box, I realized others might benefit from what I had learned. After laboring for several years, I finally gave birth to the first edition of *Into the Mouths of Babes* in 1984. It cracks me up to think the original manuscript was created on an electric typewriter. The second edition came a decade later (thank you, computers . . .) in 1995. Now, close to 30 years after the publication of the original version, I am happy to present this completely revised edition to you.

I am delighted to report that Zack and Molly, the children we raised on natural foods, are reaping the health benefits as they are flourishing in their thirty-something years. You'll see comments from Molly in her preface that follows mine, as she relates her food experiences as a child, comments on her current choices and why she makes them, and shares how her knowledge benefited the children she has worked with across the globe.

In 1997, Zack had a son. It was a thrill to hand-write a personal note to my grandson on the inside cover of *Into the Mouths of Babes* that I proudly presented to his mama and papa in 1997. Another generation was emerging to be fed by this nourishing work. What a thrill it is to have my grandson and his little sister add their favorite recipes for this edition.

It was an absolute joy for me to feed our babies homemade, wholesome foods. It tickles me today when my children come for a visit, open the refrigerator and exclaim with delight, "Mom food!" And now, as an ecstatic grandmother, it is an honor to share this latest work with my children's generation to support their children in love and nourishment.

Letters and calls from readers have been consistent in thanking me for supplying a guilt-free, you-can-do-it, empowering guide for their children's early eating needs. The biggest thrill, though, is to know the recipes and ideas in this book will help in providing your child with the best beginning possible for a healthful and wonder-filled journey through life.

All the children in the world deserve to be loved and nourished. For this reason, a portion of the royalties from *Into the Mouths of Babes* will be donated to charities so that together we can support the well-being of children worldwide.

It is a privilege and an honor to share this third edition with you. Thank you for creating the time to add these ideas into your own style and culture of lovingly feeding your baby. Best wishes for happy feeding, growing, and loving times together.

Susan Tate
Edmonds, Washington

# Molly's Preface to the Third Edition

There is nothing like *mom food*! For the past decade or so, life has taken me far from my parents' cooking, but visiting my mother in Seattle is always a treat. I peek in the kitchen and I know I will find bright red cherry tomatoes, goat cheese, rice crackers, whole grain cereals, and if I'm lucky, something tasty on the stove. The tastes of *mom food* bring me back to times of standing on kitchen chair and leaning over countertops to knead calzone dough or stick my finger in something fruity and sweet! Both my mother and father ask, "What would you like to eat?" when I visit (Thai food at mom's, stuffed cabbage at dad's), and I know I am Home.

As my concept of home has moved from Virginia to Europe to Africa to various Midwestern States, back to Africa, and now back to Europe again, I have needed to find a way to re-create nourishing home-food. My first Thanksgiving away from my family, I invited an international group of friends over for a French version of an American holiday. I delighted in feeding the group a motley meal as we all squeezed together in my tiny Provençal flat. When college cafeteria food wasn't cutting it in Wisconsin, my friend Jenny and I decided that we would cook for ourselves. Tofu and vegetables were always on hand and for those days that called for a quick mac 'n cheese dinner, we always chose organics and tossed in some green peas. During graduate school on those lucky days of classes ending early, my roommate Laura and I would chop and sauté together, light candles, and sit on floor pillows to eat my mom's lentil soup. When my job took me to Iraq, I trolled from market to market to find the right ingredients for my Babba's Easter bread. Now, my partner Patrick and I live in Brussels where the farmer's markets intoxicate you with their brilliantly colored produce overflowing their baskets—you can never go home empty-handed or empty-bellied for that matter.

I have always taken pleasure in eating, but in our fast-paced culture we can forget to savor and slow down. As I've traveled and reveled in placelessness, I have learned the language of food and the importance of sharing, eating, and enjoying it. In Senegal, I was invited into neighbors' homes during mealtime (you can't leave without taking a bite), and food was prepared from sun up to sun down. In Srebrenica, Bosnia, we were served a three-hour feast for lunch including beef raised in the fields where thyme and rosemary peppered the air as well as our foods. Being raised vegetarian, I must admit this beautiful meal has changed my diet a smidge!

In many of these places, I have worked with children in various settings and have loved sharing my mother's wellness wisdom. Working as a nanny for five, I made sure that the dinner assembly line included greens and fruits. One of my favorite kitchen memories with the children is plopping the three-year-old girl on the countertop and creating jam with the ruby berries we had picked from the family garden together.

As my childhood friends are in the creational transition to the next generation of mamas and papas, I so wanted my mother to create an updated *Into the Mouths of Babes* for them. I have loved watching my old and new friends welcome new little beings into the world with amazement and grace. I wish their babies and yours a plate full of peace, strength, and nourishing tastes. I invite you to squish those bananas, giggle in the kitchen, and marvel in life's flavors. Bon appétit to you and your baby!

Molly Firkaly
Brussels, Belgium

# Introduction to the Third Edition

*A new baby is like the beginning of all things—*
*wonder, hope, a dream of possibilities.*
~ Eda J. LeShan

Good nutrition is a lifelong gift to our children. It can support and nourish them along a path of wonder and possibility. The purpose of this book is to offer information and supportive guidance to create the best start possible as you make wise choices for feeding your new baby or toddler.

This revised edition contains the latest science-based and mind-body research to support healthy feeding choices for your child. It is offered to you through the lens of my lifelong exploration of health, wellness, food, love, and sacred nourishment.

When I conceived the idea for the first edition, I was a young mother who delighted in planning, preparing, and discovering the healthiest ways to feed our children. At that time, books on how to feed babies a vegetarian diet were scarce. When I revised the second edition of *Into the Mouths of Babes* in the mid-90s, I was an assistant professor in the School of Medicine and the Director of Health Promotion at the University of Virginia. I had an inside view of what university women and men dealt with when it came to body image and food issues. That experience led me to expand my literature review as I updated the research on the topic of disordered eating and body dissatisfaction in both the second and third editions.

A 2004 study published in *Health Education Research* reported significant correlation between parents and their children in the areas of snacking, eating motivation, and body dissatisfaction. The study concluded that a positive parental role model was more effective in improving a child's diet than attempts to control what their children ate. So I hope this next statement isn't too shocking: Providing your child with the best nourishment possible may mean it's not always about the food.

With this in mind, you will discover the heart of this edition to be the concept that nourishing a baby involves much more than the foods we select or our knowledge of nutrition. My addition of "Seven Sacred Nutrients" in chapter 6 provides an expanded framework for viewing infant nourishment. These particular nutrients can't be purchased at the grocery store, and you won't find them on food labels, but I believe they are essential to supporting the best possible nourishment for your child. These sacred nutrients include but are not limited to Joy, Wisdom, Respect, Quality, Safety, Pleasure and, of course, Love. They can be given in unlimited quantities at any age.

Over the years, I have often replaced the word *nutrition* with *nourishment*. Nourishment represents a broader and more holistic approach to thinking about food and eating. It involves the mind, body, spirit, and emotions rather than just scientific facts about the nutrient content of foods. It includes how we think and feel about food and eating. It includes your choice to make your own baby food too.

Mothers, fathers, and other caregivers can easily follow these recipes. Most books assume the mother prepares food for "her" baby. This book honors the fact that many partners take an active role in parenting. Gender-biased and stereotyped books on child rearing and feeding are unfair and do not acknowledge the diversity of family structures in today's world. With this in mind, I often use the word *parent* or *caregiver* instead of *mother*. I also alternate using masculine and feminine pronouns when referring to babies throughout this book.

Many parents prefer opening a jar and feeding their babies with only seconds of preparation. Who can blame them, with only twenty-four hours in a day and a baby taking up twenty-three? Many of the nutritious recipes presented here are as quick and easy to prepare as store-bought products. There are also recipes for preparing large batches of food that can be frozen for later use. Whether working inside or outside the home, parents need timesaving ideas so they are not chained to the high chair.

You may choose to wait until after the first year to introduce meat, chicken, or fish; or you may decide to raise your child with vegetarian foods. The information in this book can be a guide for you regardless of your preference, although these recipes contain no meat. If you do choose to add meat, wait until your child has reached her first birthday, since meat will be more easily digested then. Be sure to check other resources to assist your choices in this area.

It is important to be comfortable with your choice and knowledgeable about whatever eating plan you may choose. If you feed your baby a vegan diet, know ahead of time that this book has many vegan recipes. However, it is targeted more to vegetarian choices, so you will want to also seek information from experts in the vegan community.

While scrutinizing pages of research on nutrition, nourishment, and infant feeding, I found amazing contradictions in numerous areas. "Nutrition is a funny science," says Joshua Rosenthal, founder of the Institute for Integrative Nutrition. "It's the only field where people can scientifically prove opposing theories and still be right." And Marc David, respected nutritional psychologist who is founder and director of the Institute for the Psychology of Eating suggests, "The field of nutrition is frontier land. It's the Wild West."

You'll be given a variety of whole food recipes that can be used instead of or along with prepared baby food. Though there is no single right way to feed your baby, *Into the Mouths of Babes*, is intended as a loving guide to feeding your infant, along with your own instincts and advice from your child's pediatrician.

Where conflicting informed opinions exist regarding starting ages for a certain food, I have chosen the later starting date. Children have their entire lives to eat a variety of foods. I see no reason to rush the introduction of too many foods too early and thereby risk possible allergic reactions.

Before the recipe chapters, you will find information on how, what, and when to feed your baby, as well as what you may want to feed yourself. I have greatly expanded the chapter on prenatal nutrition, "Into the Mouths of Future Moms," and it precedes the chapter on infant nutrition.

You'll find the recipes divided into six chapters: "Beginner Recipes" (starting at age six months); "Intermediate Recipes" (for ages seven to nine months); "Advanced Recipes" (ages ten to twelve months); "Toddle Food" (for the toddling one- to two-year-olds); "Whole-Family Recipes," which provides wholesome recipes for all ages so that a natural progression from infancy can be continued; and "Recipes for a Child With Allergies," which includes suggestions for preparing food when milk, wheat, or gluten allergies, as well as hypersensitivities must be considered. With the increase in gluten sensitivities, I've added recipes and information on this topic in the "Coping with Food Allergies" chapter. You'll also find excellent follow-up resources in the bibliography.

The bibliography also contains every resource listed in this edition plus other supporting material that has been instrumental in shaping the content of this book. So, know that every time you see a book or study referenced, you will find details in the expanded bibliography.

The "Closing Thoughts" include gentle suggestions on where to go after reading this book. You'll also find "The Voice of Self-Care," designed to lovingly support you as you create your own way of doing the most important job on the planet—caring for the children.

Preparation time for these recipes varies, but many foods can be prepared in ten minutes or less. It would be wise to prepare them when "spare" time allows so that, on a daily basis, less preparation would be needed. As an example, oats can be ground in a food processor or blender, placed in a clean jar, labeled, and then cooked as needed. Batches of vegetables can be made up all at one time and frozen in ice cube trays for later use. The recipes that take a little longer to prepare can easily be planned around your family's meal for that day. I discovered it was worth taking ten to fifteen minutes to plan a weekly menu. And then I discovered I rarely had time to actually do that! So see what works best in your life. Having family members call out their suggestions to you can be of help and also lets everyone contribute to menu planning. Sharing this task, as well as the cooking, helps others in the family share the joys and responsibility of feeding the new little one.

It was a mindful decision not to include any food pyramids (or food plates) in this edition. Rather than a food pyramid, I love the simplicity of Michael Pollan's recommendation in his book, *In Defense of Food*: "Eat food. Not too much. Mostly plants." I would add a bit more to that by suggesting: Eat a variety of wholesome, unprocessed, non-genetically modified, colorful, locally and organically grown (if possible) foods in a relaxed and peaceful setting, and get adequate exercise. And then I'd sprinkle the food with the sacred nutrients you'll read about in chapter 6.

With childhood obesity being a major health issue today, your choices are more important than ever. Current statistics from the Centers for Disease Control and Prevention inform us that childhood obesity has more than tripled in the last 30 years. The good news is that healthy eating and physical activity make obesity preventable.

Good nutrition can be a lifelong gift to our children. As parents we have the responsibility to provide nourishment that will help our beautiful little ones blossom into unique, healthy adults. It is my wish for you that the recipes and ideas in this book will help to provide your child with the best start possible for a healthful journey through life.

*Chapter One*

# WHY MAKE YOUR OWN BABY FOOD?

With ready-made foods and microwaves, why bother making your own baby food? Of course, it is so easy to open a jar, but the comparison between what is in that jar and what is in your very own home-prepared food is quite noteworthy.

## NUTRITIONAL QUALITY

The nutritional superiority of a homemade product is the best reason to make your own. If you make baby food from scratch, you can choose fresh vegetables, fruits, and whole grains to serve without adding any unnecessary ingredients. Foods can be picked from your garden, purchased at your local farmer's market or Community Supported Agriculture (CSA), or carefully selected from your local grocer. Homemade products don't need preservatives to lengthen shelf life because they are eaten fresh daily or quickly frozen for later use.

## ECONOMY

It's more economical to make your own baby food! Choosing to make your own baby food can be a way to save money while providing fresher foods for your baby. When making one's own baby food, there is no expense for the jars, labor, packaging, advertising, or "extra" ingredients. The cost of a baby food jar alone often comprises one-third of the price passed on to the consumer. Many commercial jars of food contain water, and the consumer pays for that liquid weight. Of course, homemade foods may sometimes contain water, but it's your water, prepared along with your fresh ingredients.

## CONTROL OF INGREDIENTS

Many commercially prepared baby foods still contain modified starch to keep the food from separating and to act as a thickening agent. This starch is treated with acids in the process of being made into this unnecessary additive.

Another benefit of making your own baby food is the decreased risk of bisphenol-A (BPA) and other chemical exposure from food packaging. It was shocking to learn many manufacturers still use BPA in the inner coating of cans and the plastic seal under the metal jar lids of baby food. Several states have passed legislation to ban BPA from food packaging. Hooray for the state of Maine since they have been one of the strongest leaders in protecting children from this kind of chemical exposure. Fortunately, global awareness of this risky practice has increased. In late 2012, France passed a law banning BPA from baby food packaging and other countries are beginning to do the same.

Although baby food on the shelves is better than in the past, some of it still contains salt and sugar. The increased nutritional awareness of consumers has forced companies to remove some of these unnecessary ingredients from most of their baby foods.

There is one ingredient that neither Gerber nor Heinz can add—and that ingredient is your *love*. Preparing and sharing food, especially with your own family, feels good, and being able to add that loving touch feels even better. The satisfaction of knowing the food you make contains only the best ingredients is yet another reason to make your own baby food.

## DETERMINE WHAT'S RIGHT FOR YOU AND YOUR BABY

Giving your child nutritious foods that are served in a loving, peaceful manner is much more important than knocking yourself out trying to make every single food that enters your baby's mouth. It's so important to feel comfortable in your role as "nutritionist" for your child. You might be happy making vegetables and fruits but prefer buying prepared cereals rather than grinding and cooking grains. That's great! You might buy some foods and make homemade foods when you have time. That's great too! Or you might choose to make everything from scratch. There is no single absolutely right way of feeding your baby. Make choices that suit you and your lifestyle. Whichever way you opt for—have fun.

# Chapter Two

# YOUR KITCHEN LAYETTE

Clean hands, utensils, and cookware in the kitchen are vital to the preparation of safe homemade baby food. Take inventory of the cookware, storage, and serving equipment you already have, and then add any of the items from the following lists that will help to complete your "kitchen layette."

It is not necessary to have all of these items in order to make your baby's food, just as it is not imperative that a baby has six side-snap undershirts, six onesies, six sleepers, four receiving blankets, two hats, and seven pairs of socks! After you read through some recipes, use your own judgment to decide what you will need.

Use glass or stainless steel items (these can be reused and recycled) and be sure your baby's bottles and dishes are BPA-free. The U.S. Food and Drug Administration announced in July 2012 that manufacturers are no longer allowed to use bisphenol-A (BPA) in baby bottles or sippy cups. Check to see if you have older bottles or dishes still in your home that contain this unsafe chemical.

## To Prepare:

| | |
|---|---|
| Baby food grinder | Steamer basket |
| Blender | Food mill |
| Immersion blender | Food processor |
| Grater | Pressure cooker |

## To Store:
Plastic freezer or BPA-free bottle bags
Ice cube trays
Glass jars

## To Serve:
Bib
Baby spoon
High chair
Spouted cup
Heated baby dish

## To Travel:
Lunch box
Thermos
Water bottle

> **MICROWAVE SAFETY TIPS**
> If you are using a microwave to heat baby's food, be sure to stir after heating and then test the food yourself before serving. Microwaves heat unevenly and one bite of food may be hotter (or cooler) than another bite. Do not heat baby bottles in the microwave. The uneven heating can result in serious burns for your little one.

**Baby food mill/grinder.** These clever little baby food grinders are a vital necessity. Ask anyone who has ever used one—they're great! For use at home, just put the foods you want pureed into the cylinder, grind, and serve right from the food mill. Whip it out at a restaurant or at a friend's house for dinner, and add the foods you select for your baby. It's like carrying a miniature cordless blender in your purse or diaper bag. Baby food grinders are inexpensive (under fifteen dollars) and are worth every penny. Don't bother with the electric baby food mills, the hand held ones are just perfect. (Note: A copy of *Into the Mouths of Babes* and a baby food grinder make a delightful shower gift.)

**Blender.** A blender is a great timesaving appliance if you seriously plan to prepare your baby's food. It doesn't have to have eighteen speeds—any old blender will do.

**Immersion (Stick) Blender.** Another great option is the handheld stick blender. It's an easy way to quickly and easily puree vegetables and fruits. The cleanup is easier than with upright blenders. Although they make smaller ones for preparing baby food, the regular models will do quite nicely.

**Grater.** A small hand grater is needed for some of the vegetable recipes. A food processor would be a real treat to have, but a grater works "great" and doesn't use electricity.

**Steamer basket.** A collapsible steamer basket is needed for cooking vegetables with steam. You'll just slip this inexpensive basket inside a saucepan containing about an inch of water. (Water should not touch the vegetables.) After covering the saucepan with a tight-fitting lid, steaming vegetables over medium heat is an easy way to cook. There is no need to stir. Steaming (but not overcooking) is a good way to save the valuable vitamin content in vegetables.

**Food mill.** Food mills are larger versions of the baby food grinder, allowing larger quantities of foods to be blended at one time. While not a necessity, a food mill can be useful in preparing baby food, particularly if a blender or food processor is not already in your kitchen.

**Food processor.** If you are interested in saving time in the kitchen, this appliance is a delight. It blends, purees, grates, or grinds a larger amount than the blender. A food processor is not necessary for baby food making, but it saves time in many ways.

**Pressure cooker.** This timesaving, nutrient-saving device is wonderful for cooking large batches of fruits, vegetables, and other foods. Although a pressure cooker is not essential to preparing baby food, it is a big help. You may have heard horror stories about the lids flying off and sending green beans all over the ceiling. A pressure cooker need not be feared if: (1) you read and follow the directions and (2) you don't leave the pressure cooker on while you go grocery shopping.

People who use their pressure cookers love them. If you happen to own an "antique" version made before the 1980s, be extra careful monitoring the jiggle-top steam regulator. If you own one made before these improvements, check to be sure the rubber gasket is in good condition and not brittle. New gaskets are available in housewares sections at larger department stores.

Check Lorna Sass's book, *Recipes from an Ecological Kitchen* for more ideas and instructions about pressure cookers. Rediscover the pressure cooker you may have in your cupboard, read the directions, and pride yourself on finding another way to save time and nutrients in the kitchen.

**Ice cube trays.** A few ice cube trays are needed for freezing large quantities of fruits and vegetables. As soon as the cubes are frozen, plop them into a plastic bag, label, date, and store in the freezer.

**Breast milk storage options.** La Leche League International offers these suggestions for best options for storing human milk:

- Glass or hard-sided plastic containers with well-fitting tops
- BPA-free containers
- Containers that have been washed in hot soapy water, rinsed well, and allowed to air dry before use
- Freezer milk bags designed for storing human milk
- Leave an inch of space at the top to allow the milk to expand as it freezes.

**Plastic freezer bags**. These can be used to hold the various frozen food cubes prepared in your kitchen. Be sure to label each bag. It's amazing how things can get lost in a freezer. The individual, sterile plastic baby bottle bags are wonderful to hold frozen food cubes to take traveling, whether out to a friend's for lunch or on a road trip to see the grandparents.

**Glass jars.** Sterile glass jars (canning jars or peanut butter jars) are good for storing ground oats and other grains. Remember to label each jar, or you will be astonished at how everything looks the same next time you check your shelf.

**Bib.** Unless you're a masochist, a few bibs on hand go a long way in saving your sanity. They (almost) eliminate food stains (watch out for peaches and bananas) and keep your baby from getting sticky and gooey (at least where the bib is).

**Baby spoon.** A slender spoon made just for baby's mouth must be much easier to use than an adult-size spoon. (Imagine eating your cereal from a large serving spoon—good tasting, but mouth stretching!) Some babies seem to prefer plastic-coated spoons (BPA-free, of course); others are just glad they are fed.

**High chair.** A high chair is a wonderful invention. It provides baby with a comfortable place to eat and grownups with a little bit of breathing time. Be sure baby is secured safely in the seat belt, but never assume she won't slip out or stand up and fall out of the chair. The tray provides a nice place for finger foods that baby can reach for (or throw all over the floor). An old plastic tablecloth placed beneath the high chair is an excellent floor or carpet saver.

**Spouted cup.** A small cup with lid and spout top is great for introducing the cup to your six-month-old. By eight to nine months, using a cup can be second nature. Encourage your baby to hold the cup. Many children are weaned from breast milk or the bottle at twelve months and go successfully to using the cup. Avoid buying the weighted "no-tip" cups. They're often too heavy or awkward for a baby to pick up easily.

**Heated baby dish.** This is helpful and convenient, but not a necessity. A heated dish is great for melting your frozen food cubes, but a small saucepan (egg poaching size) will do the job just fine. Any small bowl can be used to serve the food.

**Lunch bag**. A lunch bag or tote to carry little food items like veggies, fruit, crackers, or a thermos is helpful to have when leaving the house. Infants and children who spend some of their day with a day care provider or at preschool can have access to the healthy foods you pack. Packing a lunch to take to a restaurant or friend's house ensures your child is eating the foods you choose for him. Cloth or metal lunch boxes work well. If you choose plastic, be sure it's BPA and phthalate-free. Remember to include a bib, spoon, baby cup, and wet washcloth for quick face and hand cleaning when going out to a restaurant or out for the afternoon. (A wet washcloth in a plastic bag added to a backpack, diaper bag, purse, or lunch box saves money on baby wipes and always comes in handy.)

**Thermos.** Inside every lunch box can be a thermos for baby's soup, cereal, or water. Having a thermos handy will guarantee your child will have a nutritious drink wherever you go.

**Water bottle.** Once breastfeeding or formula feeding ends, having a water bottle will help start a great habit. Filling it with filtered water and always having it in the car, bus, train, or on plane trips will be a nourishing gift to your child.

*Chapter Three*

# A SHOPPER'S GUIDE
# TO WHOLE FOODS

A whole foods diet for baby should contain a variety of healthy, colorful foods. This chapter contains a guide to choosing healthy foods that can be substituted for processed, bleached, refined, or artificial foods.

## FOOD LABELING

Consumer advocates have worked hard to ensure food labels are accurate. In 2012, new Canadian food labeling required manufacturers of processed or prepackaged foods to list certain ingredients that could trigger an allergic reaction. That means they have to declare the presence of peanuts, tree nuts, sesame seeds, mustard seeds, gluten, wheat and triticale, eggs, milk, soybeans, crustaceans, shellfish, fish, and sulphite additives on the package.

Australia and New Zealand have labeling standards that require comprehensive nutritional information on ingredients and additives. Progress continues to be made in the U.S. as the Food and Drug Administration (FDA) has been updating food labels through the years.

When choosing packaged foods, it is good to know what nutrients they contain. In the early 1990s, the FDA developed a more accurate and consistent food labeling system requiring food packages to contain "Nutrition Facts" on the label. It has been updated several times with the most recent changes created in 2004.

This label contains information about serving size along with the amount and percentage of the daily value of fat, cholesterol, sodium, carbohydrate, and protein each serving contains. It must also list the percentage of vitamin A, vitamin C, calcium, and iron, along with the percent of the daily value this serving provides. Many companies choose to list other vitamins and minerals too. Labels now have the number of calories per gram of fat, carbohydrate, and protein. The label also includes a list of ingredients, in descending order of concentration.

It is important to realize that labels don't offer the complete information one would really need to know in order to assess its quality. The old RDAs (Recommended Daily Allowance) offer numbers that do not reflect optimal nutrition. The RDAs were created during World War II to mark a standard for *minimum* amounts of certain vitamins so soldiers didn't get diseases like rickets, scurvy, or beriberi. The RDAs were never a standard for optimal nutrition.

In the last decade, the newer Reference Daily Intake or Recommended Daily Intake (RDIs) were developed and used to determine the Daily Value (DV) of foods printed on nutrition fact labels in the United Sates and Canada. These numbers reflect "adequate" nutritional standards rather than "optimal" nutrition.

The true value of food cannot be expressed on a label. The information I would want to know would be, as nutritional psychologist Marc David wisely states, ". . . how the food is grown, handled, transported, manufactured, advertised, cooked, served, and eaten."

## ADDING WHOLESOME FOODS

The chart on page 13 offers suggestions for substitutions that will provide your family with a more nutritious, wholesome diet. If you are feeding your child healthier foods while attempting to improve your own diet, you may want to add new foods to your menu slowly. I call it ADD ON: A Delightful Diet for Optimal Nutrition. (More about this in the next chapter.) Adding on one or two new foods a week will help you ease into healthier eating more than sitting down to a dinner of bulgur, zucchini, sesame seeds, and tofu.

## COLORS AND FLAVORINGS

Read the label to find out if these are natural or synthetic. Unfortunately, many prepared foods found at the supermarket contain synthetic additives. Artificial colors and flavorings are now known to be contributing causes of hyperactivity and learning disabilities in children. Many adults and children have allergic reactions when they eat foods containing chemical additives. Fortunately, there are choices of natural additives that include colorings from vegetable juices, herbs, spices, salt, fresh fruit acids, brewer's yeast, and wheat germ.

## FRESH VEGETABLES

Fresh vegetables surpass canned vegetables in flavor and nutrition. Steaming vegetables or using the pressure cooker will save time and valuable nutrients. Shop for fresh, organic, and locally grown vegetables when possible.

# Healthy Substitutions

| Instead of | Substitute |
| --- | --- |
| Artificial colors and flavors | Strained fruit or vegetable juice, pure extracts, spices, and herbs |
| Canned vegetables | Fresh vegetables |
| Chocolate | Carob |
| Colored cheeses | White, unprocessed cheeses |
| Cornstarch | Arrowroot |
| Double-acting baking powder | Single-acting baking powder (aluminum free) |
| Hydrogenated peanut butter | Non-processed peanut, almond, or other nut butters with no added sugar |
| Lettuce, iceburg | Arugula, kale, spinach, romaine |
| Mayonnaise | Safflower or homemade mayonnaise |
| Prepared packaged cereals | Whole grain, unprocessed cereals or your own cooked grains |
| Salt | Sea salt |
| Sugar | Honey, molasses, stevia, or pure maple syrup |
| Vanilla flavoring | Pure vanilla extract |
| Vegetable oil | Extra virgin olive oil, organic coconut oil, organic or unrefined canola, or sunflower oil |
| White cornmeal | Yellow cornmeal |
| White flour | Whole wheat flour |
| White rice | Brown rice, basmati |

## CAROB AND CACAO

Carob is made from ground pods of the honey locust tree. Although it looks like chocolate, it does not contain caffeine, sugar, vanillin, or emulsifiers. Babies who never have tasted chocolate (and they should not have any before the age of three) find a carob drink quite a treat. For us chocolate lovers, it may take experimenting with carob for a while to discover it can be quite likable.

Carob powder (sometimes called carob flour) is low in fat and offers valuable minerals. Carob is a bit sweeter than cocoa, so you need to reduce the amount of sweetener if substituting carob powder in some of your favorite chocolate recipes.

Cacao powder, considered a raw food, is another option for use in cooking. It is made from grinding cacao nibs into a fine powder that can be used in baking. Cacao is a tropical tree that produces beans or seeds that are chocolate in its raw, pure form. Cacao nibs, a wonderful treat made by partially grinding cacao beans, offer loads of antioxidants and can be served to a child over the age of three.

## CHEESE

Processed cheeses usually can be spotted quickly by their orange or yellow color. American cheese is made from natural cheeses, but before packaging, it is ground, blended, emulsified, heated, artificially colored, mixed with water or milk solids—and several preservatives—then pressed into a smooth plastic-like mass. Natural cheeses are unprocessed and contain real ingredients: milk, rennin (a natural enzyme), and lactic acid bacteria (to sour the milk naturally). Swiss, Monterey Jack, cheddar, goat, and non-GMO soy cheeses are excellent options. Choose organic or local when you can.

## ARROWROOT

Arrowroot is a tasteless white powder that can be used as a thickening for gravies and sauces. It may be substituted in equal amounts for cornstarch or white flour (both are bleached products). It is easily digestible and also adds minerals.

## BAKING POWDER

Double-acting powder contains aluminum compounds, whereas single-acting baking powder contains an acidic ingredient (tartaric acid) and baking soda. Researchers have been concerned for many years about the possible toxicity of consuming aluminum in our foods. To be on the safe side, use single-acting, organic brands. And if gluten sensitivities are involved, be sure to choose a brand labeled gluten-free. You can also find baking powder that is corn-free.

## PEANUT BUTTER

Natural peanut butter contains peanuts and sometimes salt. Most brands found on your grocer's shelf are hydrogenated (artificially hardened) to help keep the peanut oil from separating. Unhealthy sweeteners also are added to commercially prepared peanut butter. A quick stir of the jar of natural peanut butter is all you need and your family comes out ahead. It's best to refrigerate peanut and other nut butters after opening.

## SAFFLOWER MAYONNAISE

Most supermarket mayonnaise contains preservatives and additives. You can purchase safflower mayonnaise to use in your favorite recipes.

## WHOLE-GRAIN CEREALS

Can breakfast exist without sugarcoated, artificially colored cereals? Fortunately, the answer is "yes." There are two general choices.

The first is to buy prepared whole-grain cereals at your grocery store. Although several varieties exist, it still is necessary to read the cereal labels. Do not assume it is sugar-free, additive-free, or preservative-free just because you found it in the natural food section. And the word "natural" on a box means nothing.

Making cereal from grains is easy and another way to provide baby and family with a wholesome breakfast. Oats, rice, wheat, barley, and cornmeal can be cooked into delicious cereals.

## UNREFINED OILS

Organic extra virgin olive oil is typically a good first choice. Another surprisingly good choice is organic extra virgin coconut oil. Once thought to be quite unhealthy (and well, in its highly processed and partially-hydrogenated state it is still quite yucky), it has become quite a charmer in the delicious and healthy gourmet scene. Extra virgin, unrefined coconut oil is rich in lauric acid, which is known to increase the HDL (good) cholesterol levels. It's great to use in soups, stews, or baked goods. As with any oil, use it in moderation. Avoid anything labeled "vegetable oil" since the source is quite unclear. Corn, soybean, canola, and cottonseed oils are typically the most genetically modified. Canola and sunflower oil can be used if it is labeled organic or non-GMO. Oils to have on hand: extra virgin olive oil, organic virgin coconut oil, toasted sesame oil, organic and unrefined canola or sunflower oils, flax seed oil (for salads but not for cooking), rice bran oil, grape seed oil, macadamia nut oil, and walnut oil.

## VANILLA EXTRACT

Imitation vanilla flavoring and vanillin are both artificial substitutes for pure vanilla. Using vanilla extract in recipes makes a distinct difference you will enjoy.

## SEA SALT

Babies do not need salt. Children and adults do not need a lot of salt, especially if hypertension is a problem. Regular table salt contains anti-caking chemicals to keep the salt flowing freely and sodium bicarbonate to keep it white. Think of regular table salt, like white sugar, as being processed. There are healthier choices. Himalayan crystal salt has become my favorite. It's loaded with rich minerals and trace elements. And you don't need to use as much. When thinking of salt choices, think of colors like pink or gray rather than the refined white stuff. Unrefined sea salt is another option. It offers minerals that are taken out in the refining of regular table salt. Using seaweed flakes, tamari, soy sauce, miso, herbs, and spices can also flavor foods in an enjoyable and healthy way.

## HONEY AND MOLASSES

Honey or molasses can be used to replace sugar in most recipes. Uncooked honey has caused botulism and even death in children under age one. Do not feed infants uncooked honey before age one.

Nutritional awareness has caused many parents to cut back the amount of sugar they give their children. Recent research has resulted in some doubt about the widespread belief that sugar can cause hyperactivity in children. When these studies are done without funding by food companies and when parents tell me sugar actually calms their children, I'll consider believing their results.

What is so bad about sugar? Sugar contributes nothing of nutritional value to the body; in fact, it takes away valuable B vitamins during the digestive process. Sugar also rots teeth, adds weight, and can cause jangled nerves.

We all seem to crave something sweet now and then. How can a sweet tooth be satisfied? How can foods be sweetened without refined sugar? Honey is a great substitute (for ages one and older) because it is a natural product from the nectar of flowers. Because honey is sweeter than sugar, you don't need to use as much. Honey causes foods to brown faster so baking time might need to be shortened. Decrease the amount of other liquids by one-fourth cup for each cup of honey used.

Molasses is another good sweetener. It is high in B vitamins and a good source of calcium and iron. Brown rice syrup is another option.

*Sweetness Without Sugar: A Resource Guide for Delicious Dairy-, Egg- and Gluten-Free Treats Made with Healthy Sweeteners* by Wendy Vigdor-Hess is a superb book to have in your kitchen. She provides well-researched guidance and includes helpful lists and amazing recipes too.

## YELLOW CORNMEAL

White cornmeal is degerminated, bleached, stripped of its original vitamins, and then synthetically enriched. Natural yellow cornmeal (often labeled "unbolted") contains more vitamin A than commercial, degerminated cornmeal.

## WHOLE WHEAT FLOUR

Whole wheat flour contains vitamins B and E, protein, iron, and phosphorus. It does not need to be "enriched" since nature already did its job. The wheat bran and wheat germ are milled out of white flour, causing a loss of fiber. White flour is bleached and enriched to synthetically replace some of the nutrients taken out during processing. It is best to purchase whole wheat flour in small quantities and store it in the refrigerator to ensure freshness. If exposed to warm temperatures, it can spoil more quickly, resulting in a bad taste and odor.

For each cup of white flour called for, replace with 3/4 cup whole wheat flour. If white flour has been a part of your household for years, make the change gradually. You might want to first switch to unbleached flour (this is one step up from white flour since it was spared the bleaching process). Then try substituting one-half cup unbleached flour and one-half cup whole wheat flour for each cup of white flour you once used. For many health-conscious people, this gradual change is easily accepted.

## BROWN RICE

White rice is another example of a whole grain being robbed of its important nutrients. Brown rice is a nutritionally superior grain well worth the extra time it takes to prepare. Cooking time for brown rice is about forty-five minutes, but it is time well invested in providing baby, yourself, and the rest of your family with another natural, whole food. Brown rice freezes well, so make extra and freeze in one-cup portions for later use.

## Notes On Favorite Whole Foods

| Product/Brand | Purchased From |
|---|---|
| | |
| | |
| | |
| | |
| | |
| | |
| | |
| | |
| | |
| | |
| | |
| | |
| | |
| | |
| | |
| | |
| | |
| | |
| | |
| | |
| | |
| | |
| | |
| | |

# Chapter Four

# INTO THE MOUTHS
# OF FUTURE MOMS

In early pregnancy and even before the conception of your baby, nutrition plays a vital role in the creation of a healthy newborn. Future moms are aware that careful selection of wholesome foods is a real plus when the goal is a healthy baby. Months (even years) before conception, this generation of women has become increasingly selective about the food and drink they consume. Many prospective mothers are taking a good look at their bodies and wisely reducing or eliminating sugar, caffeine, soda, red meat, alcohol, and cigarettes. They exercise more regularly to strengthen their bodies, the soon-to-be home of their offspring. The coffee and doughnut breakfast, missed lunch, and highly processed dinner are being replaced by meals that provide quality in every bite. The future mom is making these choices because of the realization that she is the one responsible for the nourishment that passes through her womb to the baby. She is aware that eating well is an extraordinary gift for baby right from the start. And a healthy mom is a great present too.

## WEIGHT GAIN

One of the early concerns of some pregnant woman is weight gain. Most health care providers recommend an average gain of between twenty-five and thirty-five pounds. If you are underweight, overweight, or obese before pregnancy, your midwife or obstetrician will provide more specific guidelines for you. If you are carrying twins or other multiples, you will be consulting with your health care provider to determine what is right for you. The Mayo Clinic says it best, "There's no one-size-fits-all approach to pregnancy weight gain."

The pattern of weight gain, as well as the amount, is also important. Many women dread this "heavier" part of pregnancy, thinking they just don't want to look fat. Don't worry, though; there is a big difference between being fat and being pregnant. In earlier decades, women often felt compelled to hide their growing uterus. And by the way, your stomach isn't popping out, your precious uterus is! Many women today are embracing the pregnancy bump as a lusciously proud acknowledgment of their shifting, sexy shape. Hooray! No more Victorian Age shame or hiding pregnancy or embarrassment for twenty-first century women. I salute you! *Mama Glow: A Guide to Your Fabulous Abundant Pregnancy* by Latham Thomas provides great inspiration on this topic and is a delicious read before, during, or after your pregnancy.

Being pregnant causes a woman to add this noticeable "love bump" around the front of her body—there's another living creature inside! Breasts become larger as they begin to prepare for the very first—and homemade—baby food. Without adding this roundness to the upper and lower parts of your body, it would be somewhat difficult to give birth. This leads to a very special little human being with whom you get to share your life. A healthy pregnancy does include some fat storage because that energy will be needed during labor and breastfeeding. Baby's growth and development depends on this weight gain. Most women think the extra weight is a great trade for the end result.

So where does the extra weight go? Here's a glimpse of approximately where these precious pounds are distributed:

- Baby: 7-8 lbs.
- Placenta: 1-2 lbs.
- Uterus: 2 lbs.
- Amniotic fluid: 2 lbs.
- Uterus: 2 lbs.
- Mother's breast tissue: 2 lbs.

- Mother's blood: 4 lbs.
- Fluids in mother's tissue: 4 lbs.
- Mother's fat and nutrient stores: 7 lbs.

When the baby pops out (oh, if it were only that simple), a woman immediately loses about ten pounds: the baby's weight, placenta, plus some fluids. If you are nursing, your breasts will remain larger but your uterus will return to normal shape rather quickly.

After the health care provider gives the okay at the postpartum exam, a woman can gradually resume exercise and physical activities that will help to shed the remaining excess weight. If you've had a Caesarian delivery, your body will need extra time to heal and you'll need to take things more slowly. Teaming up with a knowledgeable physical therapist to guide your healing is a good option.

Choose activities that bring you pleasure as you add movement back into your routine. You'll need physical activity more than ever. I highly recommend Nia, yoga, dancing, walking, running, biking, or other activities that raises your heart beat and get you moving.

It's important to eat three wholesome meals and two healthy snacks each day to gently keep your digestive system and blood sugar at optimal levels. There's more on the importance of keeping your blood sugar stable in a bit.

It's also important to know that going long periods of time without eating can actually add weight because your body switches into fight/flight mode, slows your digestive system, and creates more fat. And here I'm talking about fat, not the weight necessary to grow and house a healthy baby.

## NUTRITION FOR A PREGNANT WOMAN

What should a pregnant woman eat? Basically, the same wholesome foods required by healthy adults, but a little bit more of them. When pregnant, a woman is eating for two (or more if you are having multiples), so what she does or doesn't eat affects both mother and child. And although she is eating for two, (baby and mom—she is NOT eating for two adults!), the calories needed are only about 300 more a day. Baby's nutritional needs are taken care of first, and the remaining nutrients are passed to the mother—so it's essential not to shortchange either.

And this might be a good time re-frame the word and reflect upon the emotions involved in the word *diet*, which was derived from the beautiful ancient Greek word *díaita*. The original meaning of diet, and still the primary meaning, is "way of life." A few decades ago, it seemed we turned away from this beautiful way of thinking of food as a lovely way of life. Somehow we made diet another kind of four-letter word by attaching thoughts of deprivation, suffering, restriction, and even martyrdom to it. I mean, really, what fun is all that restricting stuff? Is it doing any good? Most people on diets go off them and then on them and then off them. Here's the good news: There's another way to shape shift and you get to *add* foods to your choices!

## ADDING ON NEW FOODS

In the film and subsequent book, *Hungry for Change,* nutritionist and superfoods expert David Wolfe suggests rather than focusing on eliminating foods from our diet, "*Add in* the good foods." This is simply brilliant! We know that what we focus on expands, so if we focus on what foods we're cutting out, that's about all that would be dancing around in our brain. So, why not, and here's my spin on it: ADD ON: A Delightful *Diet* (way of life) for Optimal Nutrition? What if you added kale to your salad, blueberries for a mid-morning snack, or almonds to eat in your car? Add on food choices that are high quality, plant-based foods that you will end up craving. This will naturally push out the frequent urges for non-real, sugary, processed foods with minimal nutritional value. My suggestion is to ADD ON one new food a week. When you include healthier foods in your choices, you will no longer want the foods with little nutrient value. The body will redirect its "cravings" to prompt you to choose the healthier foods first. There simply won't be room for junk. When you begin to ADD ON, playfully and lovingly watch the nourishment unfold with ease.

A few suggested foods to ADD ON:
Water with lemon or lime
Almonds
Blueberries
Raspberries
Apples
Avocado
Sunflower seeds
Broccoli
Cauliflower
Snow peas
Hummus
Quinoa
Coconut milk
Kale chips

# CREATING YOUR NOURISHING STORY

Pregnancy can be a motivating time to ADD ON to and enhance your own personal story about eating. In fact, it's a great time to create a better story, a more nourishing story to pass along to your offspring. Are you happy with your food choices at this point in your life? Or do your food choices sometimes cause you agony, guilt, or confusion? You may want to consider creating a more nourishing story around food as you answer the following questions.

## Who is eating?

Is it a calm, relaxed being or a stressed out body in a rush? Is it a woman who remembers the voice of a family member criticizing her for food choices, or a person with loving awareness of how food can gently nourish the body and soul? You are the WHO. Bring your best, wisest, and highest self to the table.

## What should you eat?

As mentioned in the introduction, Michael Pollan, author of *In Defense of Food*, advocates, "Eat food. Not too much. Mostly plants." I would add: eat organic and locally grown foods when possible, enjoy foods in season, keep sugar intake low, and stay away from artificial sweeteners. (Did you know that Aspartame has been re-branded as Amino Sweet? Yikes!) Avoid fatty foods and genetically modified foods; eat foods that are low glycemic so your blood sugar stays stable (more on this later in the chapter); and choose a variety of color in each meal. Choose healthy protein sources. Supplement your diet with high quality supplements. Follow the 80/20 rule: Choose really healthy foods at least 80% of the time. Know what good carbohydrates are: whole grains, fruits, vegetables, and beans. I am not an advocate of counting calories, grams of fat, or constantly getting on the scale—unless you get on the scale and a delightful voice calls out to remind you of the precious and beautiful being you are. Lighten up. Stop thinking restriction and focus on creating healthy food cravings instead.

## Where should you eat?

Or where shouldn't you eat? Do not eat standing at the kitchen sink, in front of your computer or TV, in the car, at your desk, or at fast food places. When possible, sit down at a table, even if you are eating alone. Individuals and families who create sacred meal times reap countless benefits.

## When should you eat?

Early and often! Start the day with a healthy breakfast that doesn't spike your blood sugar (typical culprits are a latte and muffin, orange juice, sugary cereals, and pastries). Skipping breakfast leads to weight gain, a drop in blood sugar, and other adverse effects on the metabolism. Eating three healthy meals a day and having two low glycemic healthy snacks between meals keeps your blood sugar and mood on an even track.

Going long periods of time without eating actually can add weight because your body goes into fight/flight mode, thinks it's starving, dumps more cortisol in your stomach, and slows your digestive system—creating more fat. Eating after 7 p.m. can result in what's been labeled the "sumo wrestler's diet" since your food hangs out in your stomach while you sleep, eventually adding extra pounds in the process.

## Why should you eat?

For health, energy, and pleasure.

## How should you eat?

Mindfully. Taking three breaths (and maybe saying a prayer) before each meal sets the tone for a nourishing break in the day. Setting the dinner table with flowers, candles, good dishes (what are we saving them for anyway?), and cloth napkins is nurturing and calming. People who ban complaining from mealtime conversations tend to digest their food better. Taste your food! Sprinkle it with the spice of love. Savor each bite. Bon appétit!

# THE BASIC NUTRIENTS

Now let's look at some nutritional basics. Awareness of particular nutrients needed during pregnancy and lactation is something of great importance to mothers and future moms. The next chapter will explore the six essential nutrients in more detail (carbohydrates, protein, fats and oils, vitamins, minerals, and water) as they relate to infant nutrition. But right now we are going to take a closer look at how these nutrients apply to nourishing the future mom.

## Carbohydrates

If you skimmed all the book titles and articles about carbohydrates in the past several decades, you would discover phrases like: good carbs, bad carbs, simple carbs, complex carbs, simple sugars, high-carb diet, low-carb diet, and on and on. Carbs are not bad; in fact our bodies need carbohydrates like vegetables, fruits, whole grains, and beans. It's the quickly digestible carbs like white bread, white rice, sugars, sodas, and highly processed foods that cause unhealthy cravings and can result in weight gain, heart disease, and type 2 diabetes. We are learning it's really not fat that makes you fat; it's too much sugar (including the ones hidden in artificial sweeteners) and highly processed foods that makes you fat.

For years, a carbohydrate was defined by the length of the chain of glucose molecules attached to it. More recent research has brought us the gift of understanding them in a more useful manner: the glycemic index.

The glycemic index (GI) is probably one of the most significant nutritional discoveries of the last twenty-five years. Simply put, the glycemic index measures how foods affect blood glucose (sugar) levels. Eating foods with a low GI has been shown to support the health of every body. Blood sugar needs to stay within a certain range for the body to operate properly. Eating high-glycemic foods (simple sugars and starchy foods like white bread, white potatoes, sugary breakfast cereals, pastries, or corn chips) spike the blood sugar. This makes the body produce more insulin (our fat storage hormone), causing a rapid rise in blood sugar. What goes up must come down, and the subsequent drop in blood sugar sets the body up to crave more of the same sugary or starchy foods. This blood sugar roller coaster can also lead to inflammation.

The glycemic index is a tool that makes it easier to identify and choose foods that keep blood sugar levels steady. Eating foods with a low glycemic index (55 or under) is also a major key to sustaining weight loss. Eating low GI foods has been shown to be a key factor in the prevention of type 2 diabetes and heart disease, and also a support for managing the dietary changes necessary to decrease blood sugar levels.

Vegetables, apples, grapefruits, nuts, and some legumes are found on the list of low glycemic foods. High glycemic foods include sugary breakfast cereals, white bread, white potatoes, sugar, sugar, sugar, (!) and watermelon.

It also matters how much food is consumed and that's where the Glycemic Load (GL) comes into consideration. Multiple websites provide detailed lists of carbohydrates and their corresponding GI and GL numbers. The two resource lists I have bookmarked on my computer are from the University of Sydney and Harvard Health Publications.

Eating foods with a low glycemic index and glycemic load keeps your blood sugar level stable and supports the health of the mother and the baby growing inside. It's a way of eating that is not restrictive. Low glycemic foods are essential to maintaining long-term health for moms, dads, children and, well, for every human being.

Joshua Rosenthal, Founder of the Institute for Integrative Nutrition, offers another view of how to choose the best carbohydrates. He suggests eating foods with low "HI" . . . Human Interference. How brilliant!

## Protein

Most experts recommend pregnant women consume about 75 to 100 grams of protein per day. Protein in your foods positively affects the growth of fetal tissue, including the brain. It also helps your breast and uterine tissue to grow during pregnancy and is essential for blood production.

Vegetarians know meat, poultry, and fish aren't the only protein options. Fortunately, we now know that eating a variety of plant-based foods provides plenty of protein. Green leafy vegetables, legumes, dried peas and beans, nuts and seeds, grains, and dairy products offer plenty of protein.

And what about soy? We can find as much pro-soy information as anti-soy admonitions. It can be a challenge to decode this data since research studies use a variety of soy products (whole soy, soy isoflavones, fermented and non-fermented soy). If you have a soy allergy or are sensitive to soy, then you will obviously not want to choose soy as a protein option. However, recent studies reveal that soy isoflavones, for example, act like estrogen but also contain anti-estrogen properties too. And that's good news, since the anti-estrogen properties are blocking the more potent natural estrogens from binding to an estrogen receptor and causing harm. Even the American Cancer Society guidelines indicate that a moderate consumption of soy is likely to be safe for cancer survivors. You may want to check out the research for yourself, then follow your intuition and decide if adding moderate amounts of soy protein to your food choices feels like a good option for you. Always choose organic, non-GMO soy foods when you can.

## Fats and Oils

Since you'll find a more extensive overview of fats in the next chapter, this section will focus on the importance of omega-3 fats as they relate to pregnancy.

Your brain thrives on omega-3 fatty acids since they suppress inflammation and are absolutely vital in cell functioning. Your brain especially loves omega-3s. Our bodies can't make them, so you will hear them referenced as *essential fatty acids* or EFAs. Research has shown that EFAs, specifically docosahexaenoic acid (DHA), are critical for developing babies. DHA is important for the nerve cells of fetal and infant brains. Recent studies link DHA with higher IQ's. Two other nutritionally beneficial omega-3 fatty acids are eicosapentaenoic acid (EPA) and alpha-linolenic acid (ALA). Deficiencies in these fats are associated with dyslexia, attention deficit disorder (ADD), and attention deficit-hyperactivity disorder (ADHD). Omega-3s do wonders for mom's brain too! Many nutritionally aware care providers recommend mothers begin taking fish oil supplements up to six months prior to conception.

Fish and fish oil supplements are a good source of omega-3s, but since mercury levels are of special concern for pregnant women, it's always wise to be aware of the source of the fish and to purchase pure fish oil supplements produced with Good Manufacturing Practices (GMPs). You'll find more information about GMPs later in this chapter.

Omega-3 fats help your mood (let me repeat . . . omega-3 fats help your mood), keep you feeling full, support your joints, and can result in lower cholesterol and lower homocysteine levels (an important plus in reducing heart disease). Another big plus is that omega-3s are noted for helping to reduce cellular inflammation.

Consuming moderate amount of healthy fat, by the way, does not result in extra body weight. In fact, if you limit essential fats in an attempt to lose weight, you'll get the opposite result. Remember, it's not fat that make you fat, it's sugar that's the culprit. This may be a whole new way of thinking for you.

Although certain kinds of fatty fish are known to be the best sources of omega-3s, there are many other healthy foods you can add on to your plate. Good sources of omega-3 fats include wild-caught salmon, green leafy vegetables, broccoli, walnuts, and flaxseeds.

## Vitamins and Minerals

### Folic acid

Pregnant women need twice the amount of folic acid (vitamin B9) normally required by an adult, so be sure to ask your health care provider which amount is best for you. Recommendations range from 400-800 micrograms (mcg) of folic acid. Women who are planning to get pregnant can begin to take prenatal vitamins containing folic acid even before conception.

Why is folic acid so important? It has been shown to reduce neural tube defects (such as spina bifida and anencephaly) in their babies. This is an extremely important thing to do since the folic acid is most needed in the first twenty-eight days of pregnancy.

Along with protein, folic acid is needed to help form large amounts of baby's new tissues. Studies show that taking at least 400 mcg of folic acid has been shown to reduce the risk of these birth defects by as much as 70%. There is a growing body of research that folic acid consumed in the earlier stages of pregnancy has been shown to reduce the incidence of autism. A study published in early 2013 in the *Journal of the American Medical Association* reports that Norway researchers are suggesting a link between folic acid and lower rates of autism. Women who took folic acid supplements before and during pregnancy were about 40% less likely to have a baby later diagnosed with autism.

Best natural sources of folic acid include:

Asparagus
Broccoli
Romaine lettuce
Spinach
Kale
Wheat
Avocados
Sunflower seeds
Brussels sprouts
Legumes
Nuts and seeds
Chickpeas

## Vitamin D

Researchers are finding that more and more people are deficient in Vitamin D. Researchers are also finding a direct correlation between low levels of vitamin D and a long list of degenerative diseases. In a review article published in the *New England Journal of Medicine* (2007), Dr. Michael Holick explores the nature of vitamin D deficiency and concludes it to be one of the most commonly unrecognized medical conditions. His research reports this deficiency to be a factor in developing osteoporosis as well as other serious illnesses such as heart disease, cancer, infectious diseases, and autoimmune diseases. Researchers are also noting a strong association between vitamin D deficiency and the increased risk of Caesarian deliveries.

Recent research is optimistically showing a correlation in optimal levels of vitamin D supporting the prevention of breast cancer. Vitamin

D promotes the absorption of calcium, also important during pregnancy as mentioned above.

If you are anticipating pregnancy or are pregnant, it is wise to have your vitamin D levels checked. Clinicians who have stayed up to date on the vital need for more of this vitamin (which is actually a hormone) are suggesting optimal serum levels of 40-100 ng/ml. Ask your doctor to order a simple, low cost 25-hydroxyvitamin D test or check out test kits available on line. It's the only way to know what your baseline level is. If your levels are too low, you may need to megadose for several weeks (under medical supervision) until you reach a healthy level to maintain. This is an important vitamin and I am resisting the urge to not put this entire section in capital letters. The research of the past twenty years is deep and rich. We now know we all need optimal levels of vitamin D, and more than half the people in the world aren't getting enough. Sunlight in moderation (see more in the next chapter) is one way to welcome vitamin D into your body.

Recommendations from obstetrician's aware of the latest research findings suggest between 2,000-5,000 IUs of vitamin D3 daily to support optimal health. These are quite different from the outdated RDA levels created years ago that were designed as a minimal nutritional standard to prevent rickets.

## Vitamin B12

Vegan nutrition experts point out it is of extreme importance to include vitamin B12 in the diets of pregnant and lactating women, as well as in infants and children. A severe deficiency of B12 can lead to anemia and cause a variety of other problems.

If you obtain your protein source solely from plant foods, be sure vitamin B12 is in your daily multivitamin or that you eat one serving each day of a food that contains or is fortified with this essential nutrient. Miso and tempeh fermented with Klebsiella bacteria contain B12.

## Calcium

During pregnancy, a woman needs to be sure to consume approximately 1,200 milligrams of calcium each day. Eating at least four servings of calcium-rich foods each day is a must.

Drinking several glasses of milk each day has been a standard recommendation given to pregnant women for years. However, cow's milk is not the only source of calcium in the world. For example, there is an equal amount (if not more) of calcium in 4 ounces of firm tofu or 3/4 cup of collard greens than in one cup of milk. Excellent sources of calcium include sesame seeds, collard greens, kale, almonds, tofu, broccoli, non-GMO soybeans, chickpeas, and Chinese cabbage.

If milk is your preferred source of calcium, you will want to choose organic when possible. If you do not include dairy products in your diet, you can obtain calcium from almond butter, beans, rice or almond milk, non-sugary cereals, dark green leafy vegetables, figs, sunflower seeds, tahini, or tofu. There will be more calcium in tofu made with calcium sulfate than if it's made with nigari (magnesium chloride).

## Iron

Along with paying particular attention to low glycemic carbohydrates, protein, calcium, vitamin B12, and vitamin D needs, a pregnant woman must be careful to eat enough foods that contain iron, especially in the second and third trimesters of pregnancy. The growing fetus will be storing the iron needed for the first six months after birth. Iron is crucial in forming hemoglobin, which carries the oxygen necessary for brain and other body functions. This is one of the reasons health care providers prescribe an iron supplement (30 mg) along with prenatal vitamins. This iron supplement is added insurance to help meet nutritional requirements.

The following foods are high in iron and can help prevent anemia (iron deficiency) during pregnancy: whole grains, dried beans and peas, dried fruits, dark green vegetables, sunflower seeds, seafood, and blackstrap molasses. An afternoon snack of dried fruits and some nuts is a healthy and satisfying treat. Iron absorption is increased markedly by eating foods containing vitamin C along with foods containing iron. Since calcium has been shown to decrease iron absorption, it's best to avoid taking your calcium supplements with your iron tablets.

## Iodine

Iodine is necessary to support the normal metabolism of cells. It is essential for normal thyroid function and also for the production of thyroid hormones.

Iodine deficiency is being closely studied in connection with breast cancer. You may want to discuss adding iodine to your diet (very slowly) or the need for iodine supplements with your health care provider. Iodine is especially important during pregnancy to support the baby's developing brain.

Iodized salt has been a major source of iodine for many years. However, the processed, white, iodized table salt is not the best source available. Himalayan crystal salt is an excellent natural source of iodine. We often think of the sea associated with iodine, and for good reason. Kelp is an excellent source, as well as wild cod, sea bass, and haddock. Milk, yogurt, and eggs are also good sources of iodine.

Fluoride has been associated with depressing thyroid function because it displaces the needed iodine, so taking a look at fluoride use is something to consider. The widely touted benefits of fluoridated toothpaste and water are now being re-evaluated. You may want to check the research for yourself before making any decisions.

## Water

Don't forget to drink water! Good hydration is extremely important for a healthy pregnancy, lactation, and postpartum period. Drinking several glasses of filtered water each day is essential. It helps flush waste products from the cells and supports the liver and kidney functions of both baby and mom. Water can also be obtained from fruits, veggies, and herbal teas. Dairy-free options for beverages include high quality soy, almond, rice, oat, or coconut milk. Be aware that coffee, alcohol, and soda actually acts as a diuretic and takes water away from the body. If you feel more tired than usual, you may want to increase your water consumption for a few days and see if you feel better.

## PRENATAL SUPPLEMENTS

You already know that eating right during pregnancy is one of the best gifts you can give to yourself and your baby. And you know that a healthy choice of foods is the best way to receive nutrients. Vitamin supplementation adds an important benefit.

Supplements are not a substitute for healthy foods, but they help to bridge the gap between adequate and optimal nutrition. They are a perfect "add on" to ensure all nutritional needs are being met. It's essential for pregnant women to discuss supplement choices with their health care provider.

Even if we eat all organically grown food, it is still important to supplement. Our soil has been depleted of its original richness and toxins have invaded our precious earth. Free radical damage caused by daily stress and environmental sources lead to a depletion of our vitamin and mineral stores. In 2002, the American Medical Association reversed its long-time stance on supplements and now recommends that all adults should take multivitamins.

If you are looking for the most well researched, up-to-date list of prenatal vitamins and minerals and their recommended amounts, you'll find it in the 2010 edition of *Women's Body's, Women's Wisdom* (pages 453-454) by Christiane Northrup, MD. As a visionary pioneer throughout her career in obstetrics and gynecology, Dr. Northrup is recognized as the world's leading authority in the field of women's health and wellness. The information in her pregnancy and birthing chapter is at the top of my recommended reading list for mothers-to-be.

Choose supplements that are high quality and pharmaceutical grade, not food grade, which is currently all that is required by the

Food and Drug Administration (FDA). Be sure the supplement manufacturer meets Good Manufacturing Practice (GMP) standards. GMPs are guidelines that ensure products have the potency, purity, and quality they are represented to possess. Supplements made with Good Manufacturing Practices are pharmaceutical grade, U.S. Pharmacopia certified, NSF (National Sanitation Foundation) certified, and are potency guaranteed.

It can be challenging to sort through the vitamin maze since all vitamins and mineral supplements are not created equal. One source I highly recommend is the *NutriSearch Comparative Guide to Nutritional Supplements*. The fifth edition of this independent guide, written by Lyle MacWilliam, MSc, FP, compares over 1,600 multivitamin products in North America for quality, bioavailability, potency, purity, and safety. The top three companies are: USANA Health Sciences, Douglas Labs, and Truestar Health. You may want to explore the free True Health Assessment on the USANA site (www.usana.com) that offers personalized recommendations based on your health and lifestyle.

I highly recommend USANA's BabyCare Prenatal Essentials. You will find these prenatal vitamins listed in the 2014 edition of the Physicians' Desk Reference (PDR).

Eating well, practicing daily stress management, and adding high quality nutritional supplements to support overall cellular health and to fight free-radical damage is a great gift to your health and to your baby's health.

## MANAGING STRESS

The part of our brain that activates the stress response automatically turns off digestion. This stress factor can result in stomachaches, unwanted weight gain, and unpleasant abdominal discomfort. When you are under stress, your body is actually in the opposite state of where it needs to be in order to digest your food and properly absorb its nutrients. This evidence supports the fact that relaxing meal times are essential from the start for babies and for the person feeding them.

Stress can deplete B vitamins so quickly that it often causes a pregnant woman to become deficient in this very important group of vitamins. It is difficult to have a stress-free pregnancy, but every effort should be made to be aware of stressors and do what you can to lesson their effects. If you have time to pause to take three mindful breaths before you begin a meal, that's a good start. A positive mental attitude, healthy food choices, sunlight, walking or other exercise, and attempting to sleep will help. Laugh. And laugh some more. Pamper yourself by making time to do things that help you feel more relaxed.

Consuming sugary, high glycemic carbs adds to stress in the body. White breads, rice, potatoes, pastry, and candy will give you a short-term increase in serotonin levels and for a bit, you may feel quite chirpy and "up" and momentarily stress-free. Then comes the crash, when the blood sugar that went up comes back down again. This creates the body's stress response, which depletes your serotonin, the feel-good hormone that is associated with peaceful feelings, relaxed mood, and refreshing sleep. You do not want this to happen during pregnancy or any time! Let gentle awareness of all these choices be your guide. One small "add on" of a few deliciously sweet blueberries may distract you from the cookie.

Moderate exercise (unless restricted by your care provider) releases endorphins that can make you feel great. Nia, yoga, dancing, walking, and other activities that you enjoy are just a few suggestions. Avoid exercising on an empty stomach (a rapid drop in blood sugar can occur) and drink plenty of water. Learning relaxation breathing techniques or practicing meditation daily can help keep negative effects of stress to a minimum. If you have the support of a doula, she can offer specific suggestions for relaxation techniques.

If your care provider approves, take warm bubble baths. Lighting candles or incense in the bathroom can be a wonderful relaxing treat. Soaking in water is safe for most pregnant women (if you have a fever or high blood pressure, it is not safe), and it is also a wonderful way to relax before or during labor. You can even enjoy soaking in the tub after your water breaks, a change in practices of days past. And if you're planning a water birth, enjoy being gently nestled in a tub of warm water during active labor. Your midwife, doula, or obstetrician should be supervising.

## HANDLING NAUSEA

Nausea is often a common complaint during the first three months of pregnancy. Many health care providers recommend supplements containing optimal amounts of vitamin B6, and many pregnant women have reported positive results. Eating smaller meals more often also seems to help prevent this unpleasant part of pregnancy. Certain herbal teas, such as chamomile mixed with a little ginger, can often help to relieve this discomfort. Be careful to avoid herbal teas that can be irritating and even dangerous if ingested in large quantities. Check with your health care provider and do some reading to learn more about the wonders and safety of herbs. Susun Weed's book, *The Wise Woman Herbal for the Childbearing Years* is a wonderful resource.

## A FEW MORE NOURISHMENT TIPS

- As your awareness of sugar increases, you may be tempted to turn to diet sodas. Don't. I so rarely say, "don't," you may want to see where I'm going with this. "Sugar-free" on the label doesn't mean it's healthy. Diet sodas typically contain artificial sweeteners like Aspartame. The two amino acids combined to form Aspartame eventually turn into formaldehyde as it crosses the blood-brain barrier. Yes, formaldehyde. As you might imagine, this wreaks havoc in your brain. Diet drinks are loaded with artificial sweeteners. No studies have shown a correlation between sugar substitutes and weight loss—in fact, researchers are now investigating a link to weight gain. Stevia, a natural sweetener from the stevia plant, is a healthy alternative.

- Avoid MSG.
- Eat for brilliance. As you scan the information in the paragraphs above, note how many foods can support brain function—for you and your offspring.
- Enjoy seven or more servings of vegetables and fruits each day.
- Shop around the edges of your grocery store. That's where you'll find most of the vegetables and fruits you'll want to consume. The canned, processed, and packaged food sections can be passed by most of the time.
- Include a variety of plant proteins in your diet.
- Enjoy a handful of nuts or seeds for a snack.
- Avoid eating sprouts while you are pregnant. In 1999, the Centers for Disease Control and Prevention (CDC) and the FDA recommended that people at high risk of bacterial infection should avoid eating sprouts of any kind. Pregnant women and young children, including infants, are included on this high-risk list. Fortunately for sprout lovers, they go on to suggest that healthy adults who are not pregnant and who have strong immune systems can eat cooked sprouts if they have been washed carefully.
- It's okay to eat full-fat foods. Low-fat foods often have more sugar added, and remember, sugar adds the pounds. When you mindfully eat full-fat foods, you eat less, feel full sooner, digest the food easier, and stay satisfied longer. "Low-fat" on the label doesn't mean it's healthier for you.
- Keep your food choices varied, fresh, unprocessed, and balanced.
- Enjoy what you eat, tune in to your wisdom, seek pleasure, and be mindful of what truly nourishes your body/mind.
- Pause here to congratulate yourself for creating time to learn more about nutrition for you and your baby.

*Chapter Five*

# INFANT NUTRITION

As the wonders of scientific study surpass its previous limits, new light is being shed on many aspects of nutrition, farming practices, what nutrients are in our foods, and which eating choices can provide the best nutrition. Although it's sometimes challenging to sort out what's relevant or factual, the science of nutrition continues to evolve in an intricate and fascinating way.

Nutrition involves a variety of processes, including how the body absorbs and utilizes nutrients from food. This chapter will provide a brief overview of the science of nutrition as it relates to the needs of infants and children.

No two babies have the exact same nutritional requirements. Age, gender, weight, physical activity, medical conditions, climate, and environment all must be considered to determine specific dietary needs.

It has become increasingly difficult to sort out accurate information about nutrition. You can find five "experts" who emphatically believe certain "facts" about nutrition and five more who would totally disagree with them. It seems each new study often contradicts the one before it.

Nutrition blogs and articles elicit many questions. Do antioxidants (such as vitamins C, D, and E) actually prevent cancer? Should you use sugar substitutes? And what's the truth about vitamin and herbal supplements? Should we give whole milk or skim milk to toddlers, or any milk at all? Is organic milk better? It's easy to find conflicting answers to all of these questions. And I know you are aware that just because it's on the Internet, it doesn't mean it is true! Wise consumers are checking the sources of their information.

When researching nutrition, I turn to peer-reviewed studies conducted by scientists who are not connected with or paid by large food corporations or large dairy or beef associations. It's fascinating to read the results of studies funded by food (or drug) companies that indicate their own products are nutritious and safe. And the economic interests involved, as well as the financial implications for local or world politics, are subjects of other books.

As I did in the first two editions of this book, I carefully filtered through this research using my background and experience as a science-based health educator, mother, and now grandmother. I continue to look at the big picture of nutrition and I am always wary of extremes. I also continue to maintain that balance and a healthy attitude are essential in making food choices. Consuming too much of any food or supplement could be detrimental.

I believe there is a nutritionist within you who can be welcomed into your kitchen as you mindfully choose nutritious foods for your child. Your wisdom from the nutritionist within, plus thoughtful decision-making and consulting with your health care provider for special dietary or medical needs for your child will be your best guide.

## DEFINING VEGETARIANS

There are several different types of vegetarians. The use of the word *vegetarian* in this book refers to a person whose diet contains no meat but includes dairy products and eggs. One choosing these foods is known as a *lacto-ovo vegetarian*. Some "relaxed vegetarians," now referred to as *flexitarians*, occasionally include fish (preferably wild-caught) and/or poultry (free-range/organic) in their diet as well. A *pescatarian* eats a mainly vegetarian diet and also seafood.

A *vegan* obtains protein from plant sources only and does not eat any meat, eggs, honey, or dairy products. One following this type of diet needs to take vitamin B12 supplements because this essential vitamin is scarce in the vegan's food selection. Vegan nutrition experts point out it is of extreme importance to include vitamin B12 in the diets of pregnant and lactating women, as well as infants and children. A severe B12 deficiency can lead to anemia. B12 deficiency has been shown to cause muscle weakness, fatigue, depression, and many symptoms often connected with aging including poor memory, incontinence, and decreased mobility. (Note: I know this is a book on infant nutrition, but if you know someone with these symptoms, please don't assume it might be Alzheimer's. Normal, healthy aging need not be accompanied by these symptoms. You might lovingly suggest your loved one has his B12 levels—or medications—checked, whether they are vegan or non-vegan.)

And a reminder to vegan readers, this book focuses on vegetarian choices. You will also want to look beyond this book for more specific information should you choose to feed your child a vegan diet. You'll find excellent suggestions in the bibliography.

A *fruitarian* diet is based primarily on fruits, nuts and seeds, honey, whole grains, and olive oil. And here I would add an *extreme note of caution*: Many health care providers and nutritionists firmly believe that children should not be following a fruitarian diet (and I agree with them) since it can result in severe malnutrition, anemia, a deficiency of protein, and a range of other deficiencies. A fruitarian diet does not provide adequate nutrition for infants or children. Adults who follow this method of eating are also at risk of malnutrition. It is imperative that you discuss this issue with your child's pediatrician if you have any thoughts of feeding your children in this restrictive manner.

## NUTRIENTS NEEDED FOR A HEALTHY BABY

Your baby will grow faster during the first year than at any other time in life. Let's take a look at the kinds of nutrients needed for baby's energy, growth, and development. A healthy baby needs the same number of nutrients as an adult but in lesser amounts. There are over forty-five nutrients divided into six classifications: protein, carbohydrates, fats and oils, vitamins, minerals, and water.

## Protein

The rapid cell growth in the brain (and entire body) during early life makes it essential for baby to have enough protein to achieve optimum development. The body only needs 2.5-11% of calories from protein. A vegetarian diet can easily supply that amount for your baby if whole foods are on the menu each day.

We now know that getting enough protein, once a big issue in the world of vegetarian nutrition, is no longer the concern it had been in the past few decades. It was once thought that animal protein reigned supreme and vegetarians needed to combine "incomplete" plant proteins in order to consume enough protein.

Marion Nestle, PhD, Professor in the Department of Nutrition, Food Studies, and Public Health at New York University, (which she chaired from 1988-2003) states: "We never talk about protein anymore, because it's absolutely not an issue, even among children. If anything, we talk about the dangers of high-protein diets. Getting enough is simply a matter of getting enough calories."

You'll find good sources of protein in whole grains, vegetables, legumes, nuts and seeds, eggs, and dairy products.

## Carbohydrates

As the major source of immediate energy and also the energy source for the brain and nervous system, quality carbohydrates are extremely important to baby's diet. They provide most of the total calories needed for energy. Carbohydrates aid the body in the use of protein and fat. If the carbohydrate intake is too low, the body must use what little it gets for fuel rather than for growth. Low glycemic carbohydrates should make up about 60% of baby's diet and should be eaten in the least refined form for optimum benefit.

As discussed in detail in the previous chapter, the glycemic index is a tool that makes it easier to identify and choose foods that keep blood sugar levels steady. In 1999, the World Health Organization (WHO) recommended people living in industrialized countries base their food choices on low glycemic foods in order to prevent obesity, diabetes, and heart disease.

High glycemic foods are sugary and starchy foods like breads, bagels, donuts, potatoes, sugary cereals, and chips. Feeding your children low glycemic foods keeps their blood sugar level and is essential to maintaining long-term health. Here are a few examples of low glycemic carbohydrates your child can be introduced to at the proper age (see That First Year chart that begins on page 88):

Grains: barley, wheat, oats, quinoa, rice, spelt, millet
Legumes: chickpeas, lentils, pinto beans, kidney beans
Vegetables: broccoli, green beans, asparagus, kale, spinach
Fruits: blueberries, apples, avocados, red grapes, peaches, mango, strawberries

## Fats and Oils

For decades, fat has been front-page news as the culprit of causing weight gain. Not all fats are bad. In fact, good fats and oils are needed to ensure proper use of proteins and carbohydrates. They also provide the body with a reserve energy supply. Without enough fat in the diet, baby would need to burn protein for energy, redirecting essential protein needed for cell development in all parts of the body.

Fats add flavor to foods, help maintain healthy skin and hair, and aid in the absorption of the fat-soluble vitamins A, D, E, and K. Fats are necessary to maintain healthy brain cells and nerve cells, and support our hormones. The brain needs good fats. Stored fats are essential in maintaining a constant body temperature, and they help protect the internal organs from injury.

Most fast-food restaurants and quick, convenient foods are noted for their high-fat content. Being sure to choose wholesome foods and being conscious of how they are prepared helps reduce the worry about a diet too high in fats.

So what kind of fats should you choose for your child? High-quality fats. Olives, olive oil, almonds, and avocados are high-quality fats. When purchasing oil, look for cold-pressed, unrefined, and organic on the label.

Essential fatty acids (EFAs) are found in healthy fats and oils, and they are labeled "essential" because the body doesn't make them on its own. They are important for baby's growth and for maintaining healthy skin. EFAs are also vital for cell functioning. Your baby's brain thrives on essential fatty acids, especially omega-3 and omega-6 fats. Omega-6s are readily available in the Western diet, so the key is to be sure your baby has healthy sources of omega-3s. You will find omega-3s in walnuts, flaxseeds, eggs (from free-range chickens), flaxseed oil, chia seeds, hemp seeds, hemp milk products, English walnuts, and wild-caught salmon.

Omega-6s are found abundantly in many common vegetable cooking oils: canola, soybean, sunflower, safflower, and corn oil. Canola and sunflower oils, if organic, can be kept on hand (a switch from recommendations in past years). You'll want to avoid anything labeled "vegetable oil" since these contain a mix of unspecified processed oils. The healthier oils list includes extra virgin olive oil, organic virgin coconut oil, toasted sesame oil, organic and unrefined canola and sunflower oils, flax seed oil, rice bran oil, grape seed oil, macadamia nut oil, and walnut oil

Omega-6 is abundant in commonly eaten foods like almonds, peanuts, pine nuts, poppy seeds, sesame seeds, pumpkin and squash seeds, pecans, soybeans, and safflower oil. Omega-9s are not considered "essential" since the body makes omega-9s from unsaturated fat in our bodies. Omega-9s are found in animal fats and vegetable oils, most notably olive oil.

Poor-quality fats include hydrogenated or partially hydrogenated fats like margarine or partially hydrogenated peanut butter, most saturated fats, and trans fats. Trans fats are man-made or processed fats made from liquid oil. When you add hydrogen (creating a hydrogenated fat) to liquid vegetable oil and add pressure, the result is a stiffer fat, like Crisco. Why did companies begin to produce this stuff? Adding hydrogen provides a longer shelf life. Why are these fats so bad? They not only raise total cholesterol levels, but they also deplete the HDL, the good cholesterol that helps prevent heart disease.

In 2006, the U.S. Food and Drug Administration began requiring trans fats to be listed on food labels. Some European countries are taking steps to completely ban trans fats from their foods.

Not all saturated fats are "bad" as we were previously led to believe. Saturated fats, like butter, are greatly preferred over margarine or butter substitutes that are highly processed. Organic virgin coconut oil, which is classified as a saturated fat, has gained much attention for its health benefits. The regular coconut oil added to products has been refined, bleached, and contains added chemicals. In contrast, organic virgin coconut oil is simply that—coconut oil. It can be used in cooking and has the benefit to help fight infection.

### High-quality fats (think nature):
Avocados
Olives
Organic nuts and seeds
Ghee (clarified butter)
Free-range eggs
Organic dairy products
Extra virgin olive oil
Sesame oil
Organic virgin coconut oil
Organic, unrefined sunflower oil
Wild-caught salmon

**Poor-quality fats (think manufactured or processed):**
Margarine
Crisco
Anything made with hydrogenated oils (chips, crackers, cookies, donuts, and pastries)
Cottonseed oil
Fast foods like fried chicken, fried fish
French fries, donuts, muffins
Most crackers, cookies, cakes
Microwave popcorn

## Vitamins
There are two types of vitamins: water-soluble (B complex and C) and fat-soluble (A, D, E and K). Water-soluble vitamins are not stored in the body and need to be replaced daily. The fat-soluble vitamins are stored in the liver and fatty tissue and are eliminated much more slowly.

## Vitamin A
(Fat-soluble)
Vitamin A is necessary for growth; good eyesight; strong bones; healthy skin, teeth, gums, and hair. This vitamin helps baby to build resistance against respiratory infections.

**Good sources:**
Breast milk*
Carrots
Eggs
Dark leafy greens
Yellow fruits
Butternut squash
Sweet potatoes

*According to the American Academy of Pediatrics (AAP), the amount and types of vitamins in breast milk are directly related to the mother's vitamin intake.

## Vitamin B Complex
(Water-soluble)

B complex vitamins include: thiamine (B1), riboflavin (B2), niacin (B3), pantothenic acid (B5), pyridoxine (B6), biotin (B7), folic acid (B9), and the cobalamins (B12). These vitamins allow the body to obtain energy from carbohydrates. They also promote growth, healthy appetite and skin, aid in the digestive process, and are essential for keeping good balance in the nervous system.

### Good sources:
Breast milk
Brewer's yeast
Wheat germ
Wheat bran
Nuts
Dried beans and peas
Soybeans
Leafy green vegetables
Avocados
Brown rice
Cheese
Egg yolk
Bananas
Lentils
Peanut butter

## Vitamin C
(Water-soluble)

Vitamin C is needed by the body cells for growth; repair of body tissues; and for strong bones, teeth, gums and blood vessels. It also helps the body to absorb iron.

### Good sources:
Breast milk
Citrus fruits
Green and leafy vegetables

Sweet potatoes
Tomatoes

## Vitamin D
(The fat-soluble sunshine vitamin)
Vitamin D (actually classified more accurately as a hormone) is essential to baby's bone formation since it provides the proper utilization of calcium and phosphorus. It is also important for good teeth. Only small amounts are transferred to baby through breast milk. The AAP and the Canadian Pediatric Society is now recommending vitamin D supplements for babies. Be sure to consult your baby's doctor if you have questions about your baby's need for vitamin D supplements and recommendations on safe sun exposure.

## Good sources:
Sunlight in moderation*
Wild-caught salmon
Fortified milk
Fresh mushrooms exposed to ultraviolet light

*Here is a sun exposure tip from Michael Holick, PhD, MD, widely recognized as the foremost authority on vitamin D and author of *The Vitamin D Solution: A 3-Step Strategy to Cure Our Most Common Health Problem.* "Always use sun protection on your face, because that's the most sun-damaged area, and makes up only about 9% of your body surface, so it doesn't provide you with much vitamin D. Go out, enjoy yourself, get some sensible sun exposure, and then put sunscreen on if you plan to stay out for a longer period of time. And don't forget sunglasses."

## Vitamin E
(Fat-soluble)
Essential for cellular growth, vitamin E helps to promote endurance and alleviates fatigue. Along with vitamin C, it helps to provide protection against air pollution and is especially helpful for babies.

**Good sources:**
Breast milk
Brussels sprouts
Wheat germ oil
Leafy greens
Peanut oil
Spinach
Soy oil
Nuts
Whole grains
Eggs
Wheat germ

## Vitamin K

(Fat-soluble)
Vitamin K is needed for proper clotting of blood, as it allows tissue to form over cuts and scrapes.

**Good sources:**
Breast milk
Soybean oil
Alfalfa
Leafy green vegetables
Yogurt
Cauliflower
Egg yolks
Kelp
Safflower oil
Cabbage

## Minerals

Minerals are elements contained in each cell in the body. Although minerals comprise only 4% of the body's weight, they are extremely important nutrients because they are essential to regulating many of baby's vital bodily functions such as bone formation and the action of the heart and digestive system.

There are over sixty minerals in the body, but only twenty-two are considered essential. Seven of these minerals—calcium, chlorine, magnesium, phosphorus, potassium, sodium, and sulfur—are present in large quantities. The other essential minerals are present in such small quantities that they are referred to as "trace" minerals. These trace minerals are also essential for your baby's growth: boron, chromium, copper, fluorine, iodine, iron, manganese, molybdenum, selenium, and zinc.

Calcium, iron, and sodium are three key minerals listed here. Sodium (usually obtained through salt) is typically consumed in excess in many diets. Calcium and iron, on the other hand, are often found in low amounts in the average diet.

## Calcium

Did you know there is more calcium in the body than any other mineral? Most of it can be found in the bones and teeth in an adult. Calcium is important for your baby to support the formation of his bones and teeth.

### Good sources:
Sesame seeds
Dried beans
Green vegetables
Peanuts
Cheese
Soybeans
Sunflower seeds
Walnuts
Salmon

## Iron

Iron is essential for blood formation. Iron absorption increases when eating foods containing vitamin C at the same time.

### Good sources:
Beans

Leafy green vegetables
Blackstrap molasses
Dried peas and beans
Raisins
Roasted pumpkin seeds
Roasted squash seeds
Egg yolks
Tofu
Dried peaches

## Sodium

Sodium is essential for normal growth and works with potassium to regulate the amount of water in and around body cells. It helps nerves and muscles to function properly.

### Good sources:
Unrefined sea salt (Himalayan or Celtic)
Beets
Carrots
Artichokes

## Water

Water is often described as the most important nutrient (although authorities often differ as to whether or not water should be classified as a nutrient) since it is needed for every bodily function. It is included here because of its obvious importance to the body tissues and functions. Actually, over half of the body's weight is water. The human body cannot live longer than a few days without this important nutrient.

Babies get most of their water from drinking water (filtered water or reverse-osmosis water is best) and eating plenty of vegetables and fruits. There is also water in fruit juices but you'll want to offer those sparingly, opting for the fruit or a fruit puree instead. This water is necessary for digestion, removing body wastes, and regulating body temperature.

Babies lose water daily through urine (confirmed by the never-ending diaper changes), bowel movements (lots of those too), and also through perspiration. Vomiting and diarrhea also cause water loss. Dehydration can occur in infants more readily than in adults, so be sure baby's liquid intake is adequate. Most authorities suggest a guideline of one-third cup liquid be given for each pound of the baby's weight until the total reaches six cups per day.

A breast-fed baby gets plenty of water through mother's milk, according to Karen Pryor in *Nursing Your Baby.* She suggests the mother should drink more water during hot weather, not the baby. Formula-fed babies need bottles of water to help the kidneys in eliminating the minerals and salts in the formula. Generally, about 2-4 ounce a day is plenty. Check with your pediatrician for more guidance.

## VITAMIN SUPPLEMENTS FOR CHILDREN

Although most of the nutrients needed for your child's growth can be obtained by eating a good balance of whole foods, it must be mentioned that foods grown in today's soil are not as rich in vitamins and other nutrients as they were a hundred years ago. Increased pollution of air, soil, and water has caused food sources to be more contaminated than in the past. For example, selenium, a vital mineral, is no longer in the soil in several states in the U.S. Therefore, high-quality vitamin/mineral supplements that meet the manufacturer Good Manufacturing Practice (GMP) standards are being recommended for children one and older. A great source that rates over 160 children's multivitamins available in the United States and Canada is *The Comparative Guide to Children's Nutritionals* by Lyle MacWilliam.

Vitamins are not substitutes for foods, but in today's world they are vital to ensuring optimal nutrition for your baby. Check with a knowledgeable health care provider for more information.

*Chapter Six*

# FEEDING YOUR BABY

Feeding your baby involves more than choosing and preparing nutritious foods. In the previous chapter, you found science-based information on the foods, vitamins, minerals, and other substances used to describe nutrition. Now we will stir in the mind-body ingredients, including the seven sacred nutrients. After that, you'll find support for breastfeeding or bottle-feeding, guidelines for starting solid foods, and an overview of ways to keep baby healthy.

First, take a quick trip back in time by answering the following questions as you remember what mealtimes were like when you were a child.

- Did your family often enjoy loving dinners around the table?
- Did you watch TV as you ate?
- Were family mealtimes peaceful and playful or infused with anger and discord?
- Did you go to fast food restaurants often?
- Were fresh foods or processed foods in the middle of your dinner table?
- Did you help pick vegetables from your garden and help to prepare them?
- Did your mother or father enjoy cooking or think it was a huge chore?
- Were you told to eat more or to eat less?
- Did you enjoy a great relationship with food or was food a symbol of struggle?
- Did food feel loving and nourishing?

Regardless of your eating experiences as a child, you now have an incredible opportunity to create, or re-invent, a wonderful ritual around eating—a ritual that can involve wholesome foods, pleasure, wellness, and ease. What a profound gift for your new little one!

## SEVEN SACRED NUTRIENTS

*The deepest nurturing you can give your child is spiritual nurturing.*
~ Deepak Chopra

These seven sacred nutrients can easily be added to create deeply nourishing meals. These particular nutrients can't be purchased at the grocery store and you won't find them on food labels, but I believe they are essential ingredients that can support an expanded level of nourishment for your child. These sacred nutrients include, but are not limited to Joy, Wisdom, Respect, Quality, Safety, Pleasure, and Love. They can be given in unlimited quantities at any age.

Let's define *sacred* and *nutrient* before moving on. When we hold something as sacred, we regard it with great respect and reverence. Your personal beliefs around what you call the Divine are also woven through the word *sacred*. A *nutrient* is defined as a substance that provides nourishment essential for optimal growth and development. A sacred nutrient, then, can be the perfect complement to the basic nutrients (proteins, carbohydrates, fats & oils, vitamins, minerals, and water) discussed in the previous chapter. Adding the spice of these seven sacred nutrients to the feeding of your little one can provide a high and holy level of nourishment.

## Joy

*Sometimes your joy is the source of your smile, but sometimes your smile can be the source of your joy.*
~ Thich Nhat Hanh

Introducing foods to your children with joy can plant the seeds for a lifelong, healthy relationship with food. Joy is defined as "the emotion of great delight or happiness caused by something exceptionally good or satisfying; keen pleasure; elation." Mealtimes can unfold as sacred, joyful events where you consciously set aside the stressors of the day and focus on sharing wholesome food and conversation. Preparing, purchasing, or growing food with an attitude of joy provides the cook and the baby with delight-filled energy that can settle deep within the cells.

Speaking of cells, there is now scientific evidence that proves the physiological link to emotions (joy, for example) and their connection to the body and mind. Internationally recognized neuroscientist and pharmacologist Dr. Candace Pert, author of *Molecules of Emotion*, discovered the existence of opiate receptors in the brain, demonstrating more evidence of how the mind and body actually communicate with each other. In other words, our emotions are now *proven* to have a direct effect on the body. So, it would make sense that the emotion of joy is something pretty powerful to have in the air and in the cells. It could be a splendid gift to feed your baby as much joy as possible.

Calling in the emotion of joy can assist in returning you to a relaxed state, which is also helpful for digestion. A relaxed mama or papa models that calm and gently joyful state for your child. And your child is always watching you.

Pausing to add joy to the precious moments of physical nourishment can go far to enhance health and well-being. At mealtimes, why not call in the presence and power of the sacred nutrient of Joy to nourish your bundle of joy?

## Wisdom

*The processes of the female body are imbued with wisdom that connects you with your inner guidance.*
~ Christiane Northrup, MD

New parents are often bombarded with information and advice on infant nutrition. Everyone has opinions on what is right for your baby. Keep in mind that most of these sources—whether related by blood (Mom insisting you try rice cereal at three months) or penned by experts (including me)—truly do have your child's best interest at heart. But you also have access to a deeper level of expertise that you alone can provide. Your innate wisdom, that "inner voice," which often speaks through your emotions, can allow you to serve your baby's soul as well as her body. There's a great quote attributed to Buddha that is worth noting here: "Believe nothing, no matter where you read it, or who said it—even if I have said it—unless it agrees with your own reason and your own common sense."

Learning to honor your innate wisdom is something that comes with practice. Acknowledging your own wisdom, experience, knowledge, and good judgment can be a challenge during those first few months of being a new parent. Sometimes it seems everyone has opinions on what is right for your baby.

When you pause to listen to your inner wisdom on a regular basis and value your emotions and information from your senses, you'll find you can access the sacred nutrient of Wisdom more often. I have heard so many stories through the years of parents who sensed their baby had an allergy to milk or that baby's cry was clearly due to intestinal distress. And after taking steps to eliminate a suspected food, they discovered their intuition was right.

In his book, *Stillness Speaks*, spiritual teacher and author Eckhart Tolle offers this insight: "Wisdom comes with the ability to be still. Just look and just listen. No more is needed. Being still, looking, and listening activates the non-conceptual intelligence within you. Let stillness direct your words and actions." Okay, so maybe Eckhart doesn't spend his days running after little ones, but his suggestion to let stillness direct your words and actions may prove quite valuable in many aspects of parenthood. Scheduling time to meditate or to just sit quietly for fifteen minutes (or maybe just five?) each day will go far to assure your own well-being and baby's too.

It's exciting and energizing to honor your wisdom when you are the one responsible for nourishing a new and precious life. Read as much as you can, compare notes with other parents, gather the advice of health care professionals, create meditation or quiet times for contemplation or prayer, and be respectful of your own wisdom. The sacred nutrient of Wisdom becomes more flavorful the more you use it.

## Respect

*A youth is to be regarded with respect. How do you know that his future will not be equal to our present?*
~ Confucius

Respecting baby's likes and dislikes seems like it would be a natural thing to do. However, many adults (often without awareness) sometimes continue to copy some unhealthy feeding practices learned in their childhood. Some of these may not be in the best interest of baby. As children, many of us were told to eat certain foods or to be sure to drink our milk—and many suffered for doing it.

Children who don't want to drink milk may be allergic to milk or have lactose intolerance. Babies who spit out bread may be allergic to wheat. Babies have their own tastes too. How would you feel if you were being force-fed chopped liver or your least favorite food? Many well-meaning parents have tried many tricks to get their child to eat something they thought would be good for them. It's important to respect your baby's tastes like you would want someone to respect your own.

Pausing to give respect to the Divine is another way of calling in this sacred nutrient. The ritual of blessing food and giving thanks before eating can honor God (or whatever you call the Divine), as well as the cook, the growers of the food, and the food itself. What a beautiful gift to give our children and ourselves.

Praying or saying grace before eating is common in many cultures and religions worldwide. If your belief system doesn't include prayer, you can simply take a few breaths before you begin your meal, creating a space to call in respect as you begin to nourish the body. This gentle pausing can also relax both you and your baby, creating a calmer digestive system from the very first bite.

The sacred nutrient of Respect provides a wonderful opportunity to develop a deep and considerate connection to your baby. Don't use it sparingly.

## Quality

*Quality is never an accident; it is always the result of high intention, sincere effort, intelligent direction and skillful execution; it represents the wise choice of many alternatives.*
~ William A. Foster

Quality foods include fresh, tasty, organic, locally or homegrown, preservative-, hormone- and pesticide-free, non-GMO, respectfully treated, flavorful, nutrient-rich, real foods. Choosing organic foods may be a more expensive route, but it is quite worth the extra cost. This is your precious child you are feeding! It may not always be possible to buy organic, high-quality foods, but choose them when you can, especially dairy products, so baby doesn't consume milk from cows that have been injected with hormones or antibiotics. And please refrain from guilt if you are just scraping pennies together to get by.

If money is an issue, why not take a good look at the food in your cupboards and refrigerator? Are there convenience foods that you can do without—taking the money you spend on packaging and putting it into organic or locally grown fresh vegetables and fruits instead? Are you willing to take a close look at expenditures for eating in restaurants or what you spend at the drive-up window at fast food restaurants? Re-directional spending can result in greater quality.

Back in 400 BC Hippocrates said, "Let food be your medicine and medicine be your food." This concept is another reason to feed your baby the best food possible. Organic foods are not treated with toxic pesticides and are grown with a respect for nature. Genetically modified foods have no connection to nature. This act of feeding your baby quality foods may ultimately save money in future health care costs—as well as support your child's health.

The sacred nutrient of Quality also considers the idea of quality time. Creating quality mealtimes free of telephone conversations, texting, television, iPads, computers or other electronics, arguments, and loud noises can be a wonderful gift to give your child and yourself. It's best to be completely present to the act of feeding your baby. You are the quality control expert here.

## Safety

*An ounce of prevention is worth a pound of cure.*
~ Ben Franklin

You already know that clean hands, clean food, clean utensils, fresh foods, safe water, and foods introduced with safety in mind are all essential for baby's health. But here are a few other tips regarding safety at mealtimes.

If you use a microwave, be aware that foods can be just right in one spoonful and too hot in another. This is why you should never use a microwave to heat a baby bottle. Simply putting the bottle in a bowl of warm water or a bottle warmer for a few minutes will do if your baby prefers warm milk. When using a microwave to heat baby's food, be sure to stir after heating and then test the food yourself before serving.

Choking hazards and introducing foods too soon pose another safety issue. For example, feeding baby uncooked honey can cause botulism or even death in a child under the age of one. If you take your child to day care or to visit grandparents, be sure to tell them of any allergies or foods that have caused problems in the past. Being aware of how baby is safely secured in his high chair or feeding seat is also essential.

The Foods That Could Cause Problems chart at the end of this chapter is a good page to copy and place on your refrigerator or to leave with babysitters. Chapter 14 offers extensive information about poison-proofing your home. A list of emergency numbers placed by the phone is another simple step to take as you consider the sacred nutrient of Safety.

What a sacred act it would be to have parents, grandparents, and other caregivers attend an infant and child CPR class together. Creating emergency evacuation routes and having food, water, and medicine available in case of a natural disaster is another step to take in ensuring your baby's safety. Don't forget to have extra supplies in the trunk of your car in case you get stuck in bad weather. And of course, safe car seats, strollers, bathtubs, high chairs, cribs, and other baby accessories are day-to-day ways of keeping your little one safe.

The sacred nutrient of Safety also includes emotional safety as well as physical safety. Emotional safety involves your child's opportunity to experience a sense of belonging, of being valued, of being accepted, and being treated with respect and dignity. It means providing opportunities for your child to experience encouragement and success. Emotional safety includes freedom from name-calling, ridicule, bullying, indiscriminate punishment, as well as the threat of physical harm from older children and adults.

Making decisions to ensure baby's safety at all times is an ongoing sacred act—as well as a vital nutrient. "Safety first" is a great ounce of prevention as well as a wonderful motto to remember when nourishing your precious ones.

## Pleasure

*Taste and pleasure are essential to life, more so perhaps than we could have ever imagined.*
~ Marc David

Eating has the potential to be one of life's most pleasurable activities. Preparing foods with a sense of celebration and pleasure is nourishing for everyone. If we pay attention to our senses and actually eat when we eat, we can derive a sensual pleasure that's abundant and always present. Food can delight the senses as we take note of color, texture, and taste. You possess an incredible power and opportunity to offer the pleasurable gift of providing your little one with a practice of enjoying delicious food.

Creating time for baby to enjoy her meal may mean that the person doing the feeding pauses to enjoy the pleasure of eating and serving the food too. Placing food on a high chair and walking away while talking on the cell phone probably doesn't offer your baby many sensations of pleasure.

Guilt-free and pleasure-full food and mealtimes may be a concept that's new to you. In our fast-paced world, stopping to even think about pleasure in its connection to food may need to be re-taught. Let's face it, most of us lead busy lives. Whether you are working inside the home or outside the home, or managing a combination of the two, it's easy to think you are accomplishing more by multi-tasking. I encourage you to let Pleasure guide your choices here.

One of the bonuses of pleasurable eating is its proven effect on our metabolism and digestion. "Half of nutrition is what you eat, but the other half is how you eat," states Marc David, author of *The Slow Down Diet: Eating for Pleasure, Energy, and Weight Loss*. This is a powerful concept worth digesting fully. The sensation of pleasure creates a spark in the relaxation response, which then sets up the digestive system for an easeful passage and absorption of food.

Modeling pleasure around food and eating is truly a sacred act. Showing your toddler how to smell her food and smiling as she does this is a way to ignite her senses, enhance her response to good food, and is a gift to her digestive system.

Providing the sacred nutrient of Pleasure needn't be limited to mealtimes. Feel free to revel in Pleasure, use it abundantly, and observe its powerful results in all aspects of life.

## Love

*But the greatest of these is love.*
~ 1 Corinthians 13:13

Years ago I gave my father a spice tin labeled "Love." Printed at the bottom of the tin was the net weight—"immeasurable"—and the list of ingredients included joy, kindness, patience, peace, trust, and goodness. The directions for use encouraged the cook to add a big pinch of Love to every recipe. I have since inherited this spice tin, and it has a place of honor on my stove.

As you know, you don't need a spice tin to add the sacred nutrient of Love to baby's meals. You can add Love when you give your children your full attention when feeding them. You can enjoy adding Love when you puree green beans in a little food mill while enjoying dinner out with friends. The options are endless.

In 1996, the *Pediatrics* journal published results of a University of Maryland study on this very topic. In this study, participants in the intervention group viewed and were give a copy of a videotape titled "Feeding Your Baby With Love." The control group was not shown the video. The study revealed that the "intervention" mothers reported positive changes in behavior and attitudes that the control group did not experience. It seems the sacred nutrient of Love is proven to be a profoundly powerful ingredient.

Lovingly preparing and serving food with all seven sacred nutrients, whether homemade or store bought, just seems to make the food taste better. Generous amounts of Joy, Wisdom, Respect, Quality, Safety, and Pleasure mix in quite well with an abundance of Love. Love, the most sacred of all nutrients, can be used generously throughout your child's life.

## BREAST MILK: THE ULTIMATE FIRST FOOD

The act of breastfeeding can provide a wonderful opportunity to add all of the sacred nutrients—Joy, Wisdom, Respect, Quality, Safety, Pleasure, and Love during feeding times. What a sacred act it is to feed baby directly from your body. Mother's milk is nature's most perfect food. It's always the right temperature, it contains a blend of nutrients perfect for your baby, it is readily available (if you are) and it is an amazing way to provide mother-infant bonding.

Human milk is the most complete form of nutrition for babies. It is easily digestible, known to prevent certain allergies, encourages normal weight gain, helps improve IQ, and may decrease the chance of ear infections. Breast milk has the perfect combination of nutrients, including the essential fatty acids needed for brain development. In fact, breast milk is so unique in its composition that it cannot be replicated. Colostrum, the early milk produced by the mother, contains antibodies uniquely designed to support the baby's immune system from the start. Breastfeeding even provides wonderful stimulation of baby's mouth, palate, and jaw.

Lactating is shown to not only support baby's health, but the mother's health too. The benefits for mom are also many: Breastfeeding signals the uterus to return to its normal size faster (yippee!) and it delays the return of the menstrual cycle (more squeals of delight!). But be sure to note that it is *not* a guarantee that ovulation will not take place—and pregnancy can and does occur while a woman is breastfeeding. Let me repeat: Pregnancy can and does occur while a woman is breastfeeding.

Recent studies show a reduction in rates of cancer (particularly uterine, ovarian, and breast); gestational diabetes; osteoporosis; cardiovascular disease; and many other health conditions in breastfeeding mothers. The list of advantages goes on: Mother-infant bonding is very strong, it's easy to travel with a nursing baby, there's no formula stain on baby's clothing, and baby's stools do not have an unpleasant odor. And there is the financial advantage of saving hundreds of dollars per year when you aren't purchasing formula. Plus, a nursing mother has the opportunity to offer baby an amazing first gift, filled with the sacred nutrient of Love pouring out from her breast into baby's mouth.

A breastfeeding mother will want to be mindful of the sacred nutrient of Quality while choosing foods to provide both her and the baby with optimal nutritional benefits. What's the "ideal" healthy diet for a breastfeeding mom? It can be summed up in four words: varied, balanced, colorful, and whole. A healthy diet that includes a variety of colorful vegetables, fruits, proteins, good fats, and grains assists the mother in producing quality milk. Each woman can choose foods best for her based on her culture, her own likes and dislikes, and her lifestyle, as well as her intuition.

It's interesting to note that a mother does not need to drink milk to make milk, but it is wise to have an awareness of including calcium-rich foods in the diet. Yogurt, sesame seeds, nuts (especially almonds and Brazil nuts), dark green vegetables (especially kale and collard greens), tofu, tempeh, and other organic and non-GMO soybean products are high in calcium.

The American Academy of Pediatrics (AAP), the American Medical Association (AMA), and the World Health Organization (WHO) all recommend breastfeeding as the best choice for babies. The AAP suggests babies should be breastfed exclusively for their first six months and that "breastfeeding should continue until 12 months (and beyond) if both the mother and baby are willing." A growing number of mothers are choosing to breastfeed for the first two years of their child's life.

## Can Vegan Mothers Breastfeed?

Of course! Vegan moms or those with macrobiotic diets need to be aware of their vitamin B12 intake and supplement with B12. Check with your health care provider for recommendations particular to your situation.

The Vegan Society makes the following recommendations for vegan moms who are breastfeeding:

- Be sure to increase your calorie intake by 500 calories during pregnancy and breastfeeding.
- Obtain 4 mcg of B12 from a daily intake of fortified non-dairy milk, textured vegetable protein (TVP), fortified cereals, and yeast extract, or supplement with 10 mcg of B12.
- Increase your protein intake by 11 grams above normal from your baby's birth to six months. (The Vegan Society recommends protein intake be 56 grams per day during this time.) Protein intake can then be reduced to 6 grams above the normal intake.
- Supplement with 1,250 mg of calcium and 260 mcg of folic acid per day.

## Breastfeeding Challenges, Concerns, and Support

The choice to breastfeed is made knowing that the mother must almost always be available for the infant. Honoring the statement "Every mother is a working mother," this level of availability simply proves easier for moms who are working from home or for those who have enlightened employers who support extended family leave or worksite day care. Those mothers returning to work outside the home will need to plan ahead, pump ahead, and sometimes catch the milk squirting out from full breasts at work when someone mentions your baby or you hear a child crying.

Many mothers use a breast pump to save their own milk and freeze it for use when they are not accessible at feeding time. Others provide formula to caregivers during the time away and save breastfeeding for morning or nighttime feeding times.

On rare occasions, making the decision to breastfeed may bring with it the disapproval of a partner or other family members or friends who may not be as comfortable as you are with this way of feeding. And on some level, that's not surprising. Aggressive marketing of baby formula has been in place since the 1940s. Fortunately, most people are aware that nature has made the most perfect first food for babies. We need to continue to speak up for our precious children to be breast fed whenever possible, as they are the ones that truly profit. Breastfeeding is a powerful act. You will find great support in discussing this issue with a midwife, doula, or enlightened pediatrician.

Family members who object to breastfeeding because they feel they cannot bond with the baby can do so in ways other than feeding. And partners can also bottle feed their baby with breast milk while nursing mothers are away. Holding, soothing, cuddling, bathing, singing, reading, and playing with the baby are all important ways to create attachment and support baby's growth.

One of the best resources for learning more about the art, science, and craft of breastfeeding is La Leche League International (LLLI). This nonprofit organization that celebrated its 55th anniversary in 2012, provides breastfeeding education, information, and encouragement to women worldwide. Their website (www.llli.org) offers comprehensive information on breastfeeding as well as infant/child and family issues. You will also find a listing for local organizations (where you can access support groups and literature), advocacy information, and an up-to-date summary of breastfeeding legislation that has been enacted over the past decade.

LLLI reports the most common problems with milk supply are rarely caused by stress, fatigue, or inadequate food or fluid intake as commonly believed. Infrequent feedings and/or poor positioning or latching on by the baby is actually the most common cause of an inadequate milk supply. And those problems can be easily fixed. There is so much support available these days!

In rare instances, some mothers (an estimated 5% do not produce enough milk and *low-milk syndrome* can occur. This serious condition causes severe dehydration in infants and can result in strokes, blood clots, or seizures. A lack of significant swelling of the breasts in the first several months of pregnancy is one warning sign. If baby is getting enough breast milk, it will be evident during diaper changes. In the early weeks of life, a breastfed baby should have frequent bowel movements and at least six wet diapers each day.

Sometimes nursing mama's wonder if baby is getting enough milk. If baby is happily growing and healthy, he is probably getting the milk he needs. With the increase in home births and shorter hospital stays, most pediatricians recommend a checkup for babies when they are three or four days old. Don't hesitate to call the midwife or pediatrician if you have any concerns about your baby getting enough nourishment.

Mothers with certain illnesses may be advised not to breastfeed for a variety of reasons. New moms who are HIV-positive will need to consult with specialists before making feeding decisions. Although research indicates HIV can be transmitted through breast milk, there are many factors to consider. In the United States, women who know they are HIV-positive are advised not to breastfeed their infants. However, in some cultures, and for many complicated reasons, it may be the only choice. Due to various interpretations and inconclusive research, LLLI does not make a recommendation about breastfeeding if a mother is HIV-positive.

What if your babies outnumber your breasts? Mothers of twins or even triplets can successfully breastfeed. *The Womanly Art of Breastfeeding* book published by LLLI suggests that multiple births bring multiple blessings; but to a new nursing mother of twins or triplets, double breastfeeding might not seem like one of those blessings, at first. With proper equipment and ample strategies from moms who have done it, breastfeeding can indeed succeed. Support groups such as those associated with the National Organization of Mothers of Twins Clubs are often great resources for mothers with multiple babies.

What if your baby is born prematurely? Breastfeeding practices may need to be adjusted for babies born early (precious preemies) or with special health needs. There are many groups that provide an array of support for parents who find their first days with their newborn to be in the neonatal intensive care unit rather than at home.

What if you have toddlers toddling around your home? Toddlers can be tucked under your other arm at times while you quietly read them a favorite story. (Perhaps this is where mothers learn to multi-task so early.) As busy and tired as you are, creating a little one-on-one time for the original members of your family—and for yourself—is vitally important too.

Breastfeeding isn't all roses. Sometimes it can be frustrating to have cracked nipples, engorged breasts, milk leaking through your favorite blouse, or a baby that just won't seem to latch and stay latched. Fortunately, many of these challenges can be dealt with early in the breastfeeding relationship. You don't need to do this alone. Seek support from a knowledgeable friend, doula, midwife, or lactation specialist.

A certified postpartum doula can be another wonderful resource during these early feeding times. Whether breastfeeding or formula feeding, having the guidance of a non-judgmental caregiver can be just the boost you need during this time. Postpartum doulas provide non-medical support and assistance with newborn care for mothers, fathers, and families. They offer education on sibling adjustment, household organization, and meal preparation, as well as gentle guidance so everyone can enjoy this precious new life.

Knowing in advance that there can be challenges was really helpful for me. The week before Zack was born, a good friend from my college days called to provide loving support just prior to my joyful initiation into motherhood. Her first baby was close to a year old and she sounded ethereal as she described the joys of having, loving, and nursing her little boy. Then she passed along some great advice another mom had given to her. She encouraged me to consider sticking with breastfeeding at least through the first month, despite any challenges during those early days. I had been planning on breastfeeding anyway, but I found her advice provided such a soothing balance to the often one-sided joy in the literature that proclaimed only the orgasmic experience of nursing.

Sometimes it is uncomfortable when your nipples are sore, and the baby is screaming, and you're sleep deprived, and you haven't even had the chance to brush your hair or teeth in days, and you wonder who ever thought up this idea of having your baby suck like a vacuum cleaner at your breast. Just knowing that these things might occur helped me to be better prepared. And on occasion, they did—and I knew the problems wouldn't last but the joy would.

The awe-filled experience of nursing both of our children makes me want to encourage all mothers to at least attempt breastfeeding. Our children were breastfed until they were a year old. And a big grin comes to my face years later as I pause to recall the intimacy and profound joy in the memories of having one of my babes at my breast.

Breastfeeding has been around since the dawn of time. Nursing mothers accessed their instincts, intuition, and elders when they needed guidance. The resources available today are unlimited. If you need support, seek it and don't feel you need to sort things out all on your own.

Your local library or bookstore will most likely carry a variety of books on the topic of breastfeeding. Many wonderful books can be downloaded in Kindle version. The *New York Times* considers the 1991 edition of *Nursing Your Baby*, by Karen Pryor and her daughter Gale as the "bible" of breastfeeding. Other great resources include the LLLI's *The Womanly Art of Breastfeeding* and *The Breastfeeding Answer Book* by Nancy Mohrbacher and Julie Stock.

## FORMULA FEEDING

Rest assured, sacred nutrients can be added to breast milk or formula. Your first step in determining just *how* to incorporate them rests on a key decision: Should you breastfeed, formula feed, or use a combination?

The decision to breastfeed or formula feed your baby is usually one that is given a lot of thought.

Many mothers are breastfeeding and love it. Others have found that a combination of formula feeding and breastfeeding works best for them. And formula feeding is the primary option for other families. The bottom line is that it is a mother's right to choose whether to breastfeed or formula-feed. Many factors enter into the decision and I encourage everyone around mama's and papa's to support whatever decision is made.

If you feed your child formula—for whatever reason—don't let any nursing mothers (or anyone) make you feel uncomfortable with your decision. Part of their enthusiasm for nursing often spills over into a fervent passion that prompts them to "spread the word" as to how wonderful breastfeeding is for everyone. It isn't wonderful for everyone in every situation. Certain medical situations and life situations may eliminate breastfeeding as an option. Make a realistic decision (mindful of the sacred nutrient of Joy) as to what is best for *you and your baby.*

And I'd like to pause here to acknowledge I am aware of my own enthusiasm and support for breastfeeding, as you probably gathered in reading the earlier part of this chapter. But I want you to know I believe that blame, shame, or guilt don't usually empower people to make healthy decisions. Please trust yourself to take what works for you and put aside any idea that might not feel comfortable for your beliefs or situation. Make your choices with love.

If you decide to formula feed, do everything you can to find non-GMO formulas suitable for your baby's age. Check labels. Avoid formulas that have a high sugar content or corn syrup listed as the first ingredient. Soy or milk may be an issue for baby so do your research. According to the AAP, the amount of iron recommended in formulas varies depending on whether the baby is exclusively formula-fed or whether there's a combination of breast and formula feeding involved. Preterm infants have specific iron needs. So checking with the care provider is important.

Make a one-day supply of formula at a time and throw away unused formula at the end of the day. If you choose a ready-to-drink formula, do not add any water. Follow the care provider's advice as to how much formula to give your baby. Age, weight, and health factors need to be considered.

## BOTTLE-FEEDING TIPS FOR BREAST MILK OR FORMULA

- It is essential that all bottles, nipples, and utensils are clean.
- Human milk can be stored in clean glass or non-BPA containers. They should be dated, refrigerated, and used within 48 hours. Breast milk can also be stored in the freezer (be sure to date and label!) and used within 3-4 months. Do not refreeze after thawing. LLLI provides extensive details and tips on their website.
- It's best that baby's bottle contains only breast milk or formula. When you give baby water or diluted juice, use a cup. (Exception: If your baby has been sick, the pediatrician may suggest giving water from a baby bottle to prevent dehydration.)
- Do not heat breast milk or formula in the microwave since it heats unevenly and hotter milk can cause burns.
- Do not use a microwave to thaw breast milk since it alters the composition of the milk. Simply put the bottle in a dish of warm water or bottle warmer, or run warm water over the bottle.
- Never force baby to finish a bottle. Heed the baby's signals when he attempts to "tell" you he is finished.
- Never prop a bottle—this could cause choking.
- Hold baby close to create feeding times that are a warm experience for baby and the person feeding him. Holding baby against your bare chest while bottle-feeding offers precious skin-to-skin contact.
- Use this opportunity to nourish baby with all of the sacred nutrients.
- Be sure to share these guidelines with any babysitters or other caregivers.

# THAT BIG DAY . . . STARTING SOLIDS!

Somewhere around his six-month birthday, your baby will begin to show signs that milk is not enough to satisfy his hunger. When his appetite noticeably increases or when he begins to reach for food at the family table, your baby is indicating he's ready to start solid foods. Current recommendations for starting solids suggest you wait until baby is six months old. This philosophy is reflected in this book. (See That First Year chart on pages 88-89.)

## First Feedings

By six months of age your baby's initial iron supply will be almost depleted, so make sure iron is included in his diet. Because cereal is a good source of iron, it is usually the first solid food to be introduced. Rice or oat cereal is a good first food. Wait to give any wheat cereal until at least eight months (or even longer if a history of wheat allergy exists in your family) because some babies may have an allergic reaction if they're introduced to wheat too early. When in doubt—wait!

The first feeding should be just a spoonful or two (try to avoid the urge to make enough for all the kids on the block), offered gently, for the baby to experiment with this new sensation. Tasting something other than breast milk or formula will be an entirely new experience for your baby so try not to rush things. Baby can be fed from a small baby chair, on your lap, or securely and comfortably in a high chair. It doesn't matter whether you offer the cereal for breakfast or lunch, but choosing a typically non-fussy time of day, when baby is content, will up the odds on your baby experiencing the sacred nutrient of feeding Pleasure.

Offer the same food all week, gradually increasing the amount to about three to four tablespoons. The next week, offer another cereal or a fruit. Mashed ripe banana is a real favorite, with a nice taste that most babies will enjoy. Soon banana and rice cereal can be combined for a meal, or you can offer cereal for breakfast and banana for lunch. The amount of food served will vary from baby to baby and slowly increases with age. Use your good judgment and let your baby help to guide you. Babies' instincts are very interesting! They usually know when they are hungry and when to stop eating.

Water is a wonderful first beverage to offer babies over 6 months old. Offering small amounts of filtered water in a small spouted cup is a great option.

A few ounces of diluted juice can eventually be introduced for an occasional snack, but keep juice to a minimum so that it doesn't replace other necessary nutrients. The AAP has this to say about juice: "Like soda, it can contribute to energy imbalance. High intakes of juice can contribute to diarrhea, over nutrition or under nutrition, and development of dental caries."

A study published in the *Pediatrics* journal in 1994 indicated that malnutrition resulted when infants consumed large quantities of juice, which left them with little appetite for food. If you do choose to give baby juice (and I suggest this be done sparingly), buy 100% juices with no additives and dilute them with water.

You can decide to offer juice occasionally (once or twice a week is plenty) in a small spouted cup. Babies usually catch on quickly to spouted cups and it will reduce the amount they drink. Never put juice in a bottle since there is a clear correlation with tooth decay. You can dilute apple juice or strained orange juice (75% water to 25% juice). Choose a frozen orange juice (organic when possible, or fresh squeeze the juice through a strainer to catch the strands of pulp that may make baby gag). Don't buy baby food juices unless you don't mind the extra cost, and never buy juices with added sugars. Check labels on all juices and choose a juice made of fruit and water and nothing else. Avoid any product with high fructose corn syrup or any kind of added sugars. I hope I have made the point—these sugars are not needed! Don't be enticed by the convenient packaging just because it has the word *juice* on the box. Also, never give a baby or toddler un-pasteurized apple cider.

Possible bacterial contamination can occur and baby's digestive system is not equipped to process it safely.

Another contamination issue to note involves well water and nitrates. Infants under six month of age are susceptible to methemoglobinemia, a serious and sometimes fatal condition that is caused by the excessive consumption of nitrates. A 2005 study published in *Pediatrics* reported that the healthy infant digestive system could usually handle high-nitrate vegetables like spinach, beets, broccoli, and carrots when introduced *after* baby's six-month birthday. However, the AAP cautiously suggests waiting until baby is eight months old before introducing homemade baby foods made from leafy vegetables like spinach, cabbage, and kale. The most common nitrate exposure for infants is from well water that has a high nitrate contamination. If you have a newborn and use well water, the sacred nutrient of Safety is one to keep in mind here. It's wise to get your water tested if you are not using filtered water.

Symptoms of methemoglobinemia include a blue tint of the skin, especially around the eyes and mouth (commonly referred to as Blue Baby Syndrome), shortness of breath, vomiting, and diarrhea. A baby with these symptoms needs urgent medical care immediately. Nitrate poisoning in infants is most often the result of contaminated ground water that has been added to infant formula.

## Six to Seven Months

Gradually introduce a variety of fruits and cereals over a two-month period. Avocados, bananas, cooked apples, pears, peaches, papaya, and apricots are good fruits to choose. Check the recipe section for preparation. Baby should eat cooked fruits until she is about nine months old. This eliminates the possibility of bacterial contamination that an infant's digestive system is not yet prepared to handle.

All foods should be pureed and portions kept small. Start with one meal a day the first few weeks, then gradually go to two meals. Keep in mind your child's individual needs, watch for signs of hunger, and avoid overfeeding. It is especially important to offer only one new food per week. That way, if any allergic reactions should occur (be on the watch for rash, diarrhea, or irritability), you can more easily identify the source.

At around seven or eight months, you may want to consider adding whole milk yogurt to your baby's menu. Babies will need the full-fat version, without artificial sweeteners. Yogurt is a nutritious food highly noted for its abundance of B vitamins and for its beneficial effects on the digestive system. It is interesting to note that this whole milk product is usually tolerated very well at this age, although whole milk itself is not recommended for a baby before age one. The reason is this: The fermenting process of the milk breaks down the lactose (milk sugar) into lactic acid. Therefore, that step in the digestive process is already completed by the time it reaches the stomach, making yogurt more acceptable to a baby who might have milk intolerance. Milk intolerance can cause abdominal discomfort, bloating, diarrhea, and gas.

If you suspect your child has a milk *allergy* (rather than milk intolerance), yogurt should *not* be given. The symptoms of a milk allergy are more severe than those of milk intolerance. They include gas, bloating, diarrhea, vomiting, constipation, skin rash or hives, stuffy or runny nose, wheezing, coughing, and poor growth. Foods containing milk and milk products need to be avoided. If you suspect your child has a milk allergy or intolerance, get advice from your health care provider. More information on food allergies is available in chapter 7.

If you are interested in making your own yogurt, you may want to invest in a yogurt maker. You can make several containers of yogurt with very little time, effort, or expense. Or you can simply choose high quality yogurt from the supermarket; but be sure to avoid added sugars.

At around seven months, mild vegetables like carrots, green beans, peas, and squash can be introduced (one a week, of course). Fresh, cooked vegetables will provide generous amounts of vitamins and minerals, and it's easy to give baby a portion of fresh vegetables any time the family is eating them. Just puree them in the blender or baby food grinder. You can also choose to prepare larger batches of vegetables and freeze them in ice cube trays for easy use later. More grain cereals can be introduced at around seven months of age. Try millet or barley cereal (barley does contain gluten) and again, hold off on the wheat to avoid any allergic reactions. If you or other family members are concerned about allergies, you'll want to stick with gluten-free grains like rice, millet, amaranth, and quinoa.

## Eight to Eleven Months

At eight to nine months, baby begins to see a lot of options. Your baby can usually tolerate cooked egg yolks at this age. But don't feed him the egg whites until at least a year old since many babies have allergic reactions if they eat them too soon. Eggs provide excellent nutrients, including protein, fat, and iron, although they are not an essential part of a diet.

Eggs are not the cholesterol-laden demons we once thought they were. According to the *Harvard Heart Letter*, one egg contains 6 grams of protein as well as some healthful unsaturated fats. They are a good source of choline (linked to supporting memory function) and lutein and zeaxanthin, (thought to protect against vision loss).

Tofu can be mashed and offered at this time too. Stronger vegetables such as broccoli or kale can be cooked and then pureed for baby right at the table in the baby food grinder.

Nine months and a few teeth later, foods can be a bit lumpier and the variety in the food groups broadens. Dried beans (garbanzo, lentils, pinto, soy, etc.) can be cooked, mashed, and given to baby. Treat your growing connoisseur to tiny bite-size pieces of soft foods too. The ten-month-old child often enjoys mild-tasting pieces of natural cheeses. Be sure to avoid artificially made or colored cheeses. The culturing process of cheese makes the milk protein easier to digest than whole milk. (A reminder here to hold off until at least a year to introduce whole milk.)

You may want to put a plastic tablecloth under the high chair for a while and don't worry about the mess your baby makes at this time.

Many people get into the habit of never allowing their baby to feed himself or make a mess trying. This is what we're here for: One of our jobs is to let our babies have success and failures! They'll never learn to eat until we let them try, slop, and spill. I'm not advocating letting your two-year-old daughter finger paint on her tray with applesauce, but it is important that we give a nine-month-old the chance to reach his mouth. Give him a spoon—let him try.

Without sounding contradictory, it is important to remember that sometimes our children sense we are preparing them for great independence. They go through spells when they really prefer to have Mommy or Daddy literally spoon-feed them. On this matter—indulge! They are just testing to see if we still will take that time with them. They sometimes seem to be saying they need that special attention. Someone once said, "They're only young once."

## Baby's First Birthday

As more teeth emerge and the chances for allergies decrease, baby's menu options can expand. The recipe chapters should provide you with a helpful guide.

Bulgur, wheat cereal, and more juices (grape, grapefruit, apricot) can be introduced after baby's first birthday. Diluting juices is still a good idea since babies don't need to fill up on the sweet taste that might cause a decrease in the consumption of more nutrient-dense foods. And once or twice a week with juices is still plenty.

Peanut butter can be mashed with banana and mixed with formula or breast milk. Be sure the mixture is very thin to prevent gagging. Also, be sure not to skimp on healthy fats during the first two years. Baby needs healthy fat at this stage of growth and development. (See chapter 5.)

## Milk Options after Breastfeeding or Formula Feeding

Various milk options are available, although none of these are a substitute for breast milk or formula: coconut, goat's, hemp, rice, or almond milk can be added in a timeline recommended by your child's pediatrician.

Choose milks with no additives or make your own almond or hemp milk. (You'll find recipes in chapter 11.) Organic, non-GMO soy milk may be recommended in moderation for infants or anyone without soy allergies. The suggested starting age for all of these options varies considerably from source to source, so check with the pediatrician when necessary.

Cow's milk was made for cows and is not always easy for human bodies to digest. With the increase in lactose intolerance and milk allergies, I would suggest waiting as long as you can before introducing cow's milk—if at all. There are many good sources of calcium. You can refer to chapters 4 and 5 for more information.

## A BASIC PHILOSOPHY OF FEEDING

Each of us has our likes and dislikes—and so do babies. By keeping this in mind and making mealtimes as relaxed as possible, your baby will enjoy feeding times and so will you.

Never force your baby (or older child) to eat a certain food or even a certain amount of food. (This is where the sacred nutrient of Respect can be added.) Babies are quite intelligent and instinctive about what they need to eat. As long as an array of wholesome food is available for your baby to choose from, he should do just fine. There are parents who hated the fact that they were forced to eat particular foods when they were little, but find themselves doing the same thing to their children. This cycle needs to be broken—for everyone's sake.

Be prepared for babies' tastes to change. Just when you think Kate has formed a lifelong love affair with peas, the next day she'll refuse to eat them. Don't hassle. Don't panic. Quietly set them aside and offer peas again a few days later.

Relax and enjoy baby's mealtime. Don't force your baby to eat. Respect your baby's tastes, as you would have someone respect yours. Mealtimes will be more pleasurable for everyone.

## Influence of Grandparents

Just as you are learning to be a good parent, many parents are working hard to be good grandparents. In their own way of trying to help you, grandparents may often want to share their ideas on feeding and may seem upset or bewildered that you may be choosing a "different" way to feed your baby.

Breastfeeding is a great example. Grandmothers who made the choice to bottle feed their children may be appalled that someone would want to be "bothered" with breastfeeding. To some it is even embarrassing. If you have chosen to breastfeed, keep in mind that many grandmothers may remain influenced by their mothers who experienced a great media blitz that convinced them that formula was better than breast milk and much more convenient. (Some were actually told that a good "modern" mother feeds her baby formula if she wants him to grow big and strong!) So it may still be a shock or surprise when a daughter decides to breastfeed. "Are you sure she's getting enough to eat?" "How do you know how many ounces she drank?" "She's crying—see there, she's still hungry." Many a well-meaning grandparent has been known to utter these words. If you are truly comfortable and confident in your decision to breastfeed or to feed your baby a vegetarian diet, let all these comments go over your head. Getting angry or defensive doesn't help. A quiet, peaceful response to the questions will go much further to keep family peace.

And if you have chosen to formula-feed and your mom (or mother-in-law) is distraught because she wanted you to experience breastfeeding, know that you have made choices that are right for you in your situation.

This also holds true for the type of food you choose to give your baby. Pre-packaged, processed, longer shelf-life foods first appeared as such wonderful new inventions in days past. And for many families, it wasn't a meal if meat wasn't on the table. Your parents fed you the best way they knew how, just as you will choose to feed your baby the most nutritious foods you can with the knowledge available to you today. Fortunately, the wealth of research that documents the ill effects of too much sugar, fatty meat, unhealthy saturated fats, white flour, and processed foods is now mainstream information.

So remember that grandparents may, at first, feel a bit uncomfortable with your knowledge and different ideas about baby food. A calm and frank discussion of how you made your decisions about feeding and how your parents (or friends) made theirs might ease any tension. Also, a quiet "thank you" might be nice to the parents who have given wholehearted support for the important decisions you are making on how you are choosing to feed your baby.

## Maintaining Balance

A word here about deviating from an entirely natural, unprocessed, whole foods diet. We tried as hard as we could to plan, cook, and provide healthy meals and snacks for our children. However, as our children grew, we came to realize that we did not have total control over what went into the mouths of our babes every day. While doing our best to have wholesome food in our kitchen, we learned not to get hysterical if our child enjoyed a sugary cupcake or a piece of candy at a birthday party in school. Our belief was that if we made these foods forbidden, we were setting our children up for being tempted, to feel guilty, or to feel like a failure. Children cannot possibly comply with this expectation all the time. Therefore, we led by example as we gently educated our children on the topics of fresh foods, protein sources, the hazards of sugary processed food, and the differences between healthy food and food with little nutritional value. Since this was what we had available at home, words were rarely necessary. Good healthy food was the norm.

We allowed some "junk" food some of the time. But it was never offered as a reward for good behavior—that would have sent mixed messages since we told them to eat good food because we cared about their health. Those times were infrequent and our goal was to achieve good balance in our daily meals. In other words, we believed a little bit of non-perfect food was not going to hurt in the overall view of things. But if a child has diabetes, celiac disease, hypoglycemia, or is hyperactive, or has some other suspected or diagnosed medical problem, those deviations from an excellent diet would be too risky and not worth the price the child would pay. As a parent, you need to make the choices and educate your child according to your lifestyle, culture, and beliefs.

As the mother of two healthy (and amazing) adult children, I can look back and say this philosophy worked well. Today, both Zack and Molly *choose* to eat a variety of wholesome foods. They still reach for the veggie platter more than they reach for the junk food at parties. I am proud of their food choices, their attitudes, and knowledge about nourishment. And I love it when they phone me to ask for a recipe! And I sense they enjoy it when I ask them for one of their recipes too. They continue to be my best teachers.

## KEEPING BABY HEALTHY

Maintaining your baby's health is a responsibility that has an impact far beyond the toddler years. Your child will learn quite a bit by copying what you do. If you choose foods that are wholesome and maintain a pleasurable outlook on nourishing your mind and body, chances are your child will revel in healthy attitudes that reach into adulthood.

If you would like to make healthier choices, having a baby is a great incentive to set new intentions. Let's take a look at a few important issues you will want to be aware of as you make your decisions: stress and digestion, childhood obesity, disordered eating and body dissatisfaction, and establishing good habits.

### Stress and Digestion

As you read in chapter 4, stress slows or even shuts down the digestive system, and there is a direct link that now clearly connects chronic stress to unwanted weight gain.

When the part of our brain that activates stress automatically turns off digestion, this can result in stomachaches, weight gain, and unpleasant abdominal discomfort. This evidence supports the fact that relaxing meal times are essential from the start for babies and for the person feeding them.

## Childhood Obesity

Overfeeding an infant should not be considered a sign of our affection. Unfortunately, overweight babies often become overweight adults. Adults with weight problems would certainly wish they did not have the number of fat cells they've had since childhood. Fat cells created during infancy (and some authorities believe more develop during adolescence) are present in the same number later in life. In other words, once fat cells develop, their numbers never decrease. This number of fat cells determines the amount of fat stored in the body, making adult weight loss much more difficult.

According to the Centers for Disease Control and Prevention, obesity among adults has risen significantly in the past 20 years. (At the same time there has been a significant rise in diet soda, sugar, and high fructose syrup consumption.) The National Center for Health Statistics reports that 30% of adults in the United States are obese. The number of overweight children has tripled since 1980. Approximately 16% of children and teens (ages 6-19) are considered overweight. The numbers in Canada also reflect an increase. The 2004 Canadian Community Health Survey reports 23.1% of adults (5.5 million) are obese.

Obesity can be a numbers game and the overweight children are the losers on the scale. Let's look at these numbers. An infant is born with 5 to 6 billion fat cells. Typically, these cells multiply to 30 to 40 billion by adulthood. Overeating combined with little physical activity can cause fat cells to increase in number. Therefore, an obese adult who was overweight as a child might end up with 80 to 120 billion fat cells. Although these fat cells are of normal size, there are far too many of them. In contrast, if a person gains weight as an adult, the fat cells already in existence grow larger but their numbers stay constant. Overweight adults who were overweight children often find it challenging to reduce their weight permanently. It can be done if the intention is followed up with a concrete and steady plan of action. Low glycemic food choices and exercise is key.

The number of fat cells present in overweight children will never decrease. Eating less food and getting more exercise (expending calories) can cause some of this fat to burn up, and it also reduces the *size* of the fat cells, but the *number* of fat cells will remain stable, making it difficult (but not impossible) to keep off extra weight.

The role of breastfeeding and its connection to obesity in later life was the topic of The United States Breastfeeding Committee 2003 position statement: "In keeping with the deep concern about increases in childhood obesity in the United States, the United States Breastfeeding Committee wishes to emphasize that breastfeeding, especially exclusive breastfeeding for the first 6 months of life and extended breastfeeding into the toddler years, may exert a small but positive influence in reducing the risk for obesity in childhood and later in life and thereby be of considerable importance in the role of nutrition in public health."

As parents, we must do all we can to avoid overfeeding and under-exercising our children. Don't put food in baby's mouth every time he cries. Let baby explore the world around him with you there for safety. Keep "confined time" to a minimum. Babies should not spend most of their day in a playpen or baby seat. Remember that overfeeding is not a sign of love. Keep baby active and well fed but not *overfed*. We must not let today's children become the super-sized generation.

## Disordered Eating and Body Dissatisfaction

Early negative messages about food can lead to body dissatisfaction for children. Not so long ago children began to worry about their body image when they became teenagers; now many eight- and nine-year-olds and even some preschool children express disgust at their body image. Studies show many have already tried dieting. Some of these children are well on their way to major eating disorders such as anorexia nervosa (starving and excessive weight loss), bulimia nervosa (binging food secretly followed by purging), or binge-eating disorder (compulsive eating).

What does all this have to do with infant nourishment? Some of us learned many negative lessons about food when we were young. We may have learned to associate certain foods as being "bad." As adults we have heard, "Oh, that chocolate mousse looks sinful," and we may have felt guilty as we reached for a second helping of dessert. This has set up many of us for negative thoughts and attitudes about our food, weight, and body image. These attitudes can be passed along to our children if we aren't careful. Adding the sacred nutrients of Love and Respect here can be helpful as we are loving our bodies, taking care of them, respecting them, and teaching our children to do the same.

And what has the media done to our negative thinking about body dissatisfaction? Plenty! Next time you're in the grocery store checkout line, scan the topics on the magazine covers. "Lose twelve pounds in two weeks," "Exercise for the perfect body," "He'll love you more after this diet," "Makeup tricks to make you look glamorous," or "Look thin in your swimsuit by following this surefire diet." In between these stories we see ten new sugar-filled dessert recipes, pages of picture-perfect models, numerous ads for drugs for every ill, and then an article on how to increase our self-esteem. And the gorgeous face on the front cover beams up at us from a photograph altered with special effects that have made every pimple, flaw, and pore disappear. Our self-esteem may take a nosedive before we unload the grocery cart.

Early messages from parents are often a repeat of what was said by their parents. "Eat all your carrots or you can't go out to play," "Don't eat too much ice cream, do you want to end up fat like your aunt?" "You're a bad girl—you didn't eat everything on your plate." "If you don't eat all your broccoli you can't go to the movies." These messages combined with what our children see on TV ("Use Thin Fast; I lost twelve pounds in two weeks") and the cultural norm that thin is in, is literally killing some of our children. Seven-year-old girls are already dieting seriously and many have some sort of disordered eating habits. The American Psychiatric Association reports that eating disorders affect some several million people at any given time; most of them are females between the ages of 12 and 35. But eating disorders are not limited to females. The National Eating Disorders Association informs us that more than a million men and boys are battling eating disorders every day.

If you found yourself feeling a bit guilty when you read this section, throw your guilt out of the window and keep reading. No need to "do" blame, shame, or guilt anymore! What we have experienced in the past has helped shape our present attitudes and beliefs about foods, but our past experience doesn't need to dictate our decisions for today or tomorrow. You can decide today to make choices that contribute to bringing more joy and vitality into your body, mind, and spirit. By learning to be sensitive to what you say, and what you model to your children from this day forward, you can help lead them and yourself to a healthier lifestyle. Your children can be gifts in many ways.

For readers who struggle with weight problems, here is a suggestion— focus on where you want to be, not where you are. If you keep thinking about weight, then your heaviness becomes your center of attention. If you focus on shape-shifting and great health, the actions you choose will take you closer to that vision unfolding.

Dr. Christiane Northup, women's health expert and the *New York Times* bestselling author, recently wrote her first children's book, *Beautiful Girl*. It is a treasure of a book that carries a simple and profound message for girls, written to assist them in valuing the wonder and uniqueness of their bodies. It is for girls of all ages to remind them of the power within that often becomes lost in the message of food, fashion, and societal messages. It's a perfect bedtime book I would highly suggest reading to your daughter.

For males and females looking for quality resources to spark and sustain the goodness in your own eating habits, I highly recommend Marc David's book, *The Slow Down Diet: Eating for Pleasure, Energy, and Weight Loss.* It is one of the most valuable books I have ever read on this topic. He does not propose a new kind of diet, but rather a supportive, well-researched, and soul-filled guide to understanding food, our choices, how we eat, and what we eat. David, founder of the Institute for the Psychology of Eating, is a nutritionist with a master's degree in the psychology of eating and infuses his wisdom with many years of experience.

The other books at the top of my list include: *A Course in Weight Loss: 21 Spiritual Lessons for Surrendering Your Weight Forever* by Marianne Williamson; *Creating the Body Your Soul Desires* by Dr. Karen Wolfe and Dr. Deborah Kern; *Accidentally Overweight* by Dr. Libby Weaver; and *Integrative Nutrition: Feed Your Hunger for Health & Happiness* by Joshua Rosenthal. And oh, yes, my book *Wellness Wisdom: 31 Ways to Nourish Your Mind, Body, & Spirit.*

## Establishing Good Habits

The overall selection of foods is also important to keep in mind when menu-planning. Adding the sacred nutrients to a variety of wholesome foods can provide your child with optimum nutrition. Any single food consumed in excess, even if it is thought to be a superfood or the most nutritious food in the world, can result in metabolic imbalance and could affect the growth of children.

Establishing good eating habits and good fitness habits at an early age will help your children get off to a good, healthy start in life. Exercise (I like to call it *movement*) is important to all of us, but especially our young. That's when they'll pick up lifelong habits. Walk, run, dance, swim, jump, skip, and stretch with your child. Enjoy yoga, Nia, or biking with them. The rewards are endless.

# *That First Year . . .*
## A Timetable for Introducing Solid Foods*

| FOOD | 6 months | 7 | 8 | 9 | 10 | 11 | 12 |
|------|----------|---|---|---|----|----|----|
| Applesauce | ● | | | | | | |
| Avocado | ● | | | | | | |
| Banana | ● | | | | | | |
| Barley | ● | | | | | | |
| Berries[1] | | | | | | | ● |
| Broccoli | | | | | ● | | |
| Bulgur | | | | | ● | | |
| Cabbage | | | | | | | ● |
| Carrots | | ● | | | | | |
| Cheese | | | | | ● | | |
| Cottage cheese | | | | | ● | | |
| Egg whites | | | | | | | ● |
| Egg yolks | | | ● | | | | |
| Green beans | | ● | | | | | |
| Honey[2] (uncooked) | | | | | | | ● |
| Kale | | | ● | | | | |
| Legumes | | | | ● | | | |

| FOOD | 6 months | 7 | 8 | 9 | 10 | 11 | 12 |
|---|---|---|---|---|---|---|---|
| Milk (cow's)[3] | | | | | | | ● |
| Nuts & seeds (whole) | | | | | | | ● |
| Oats | ● | | | | | | |
| Orange juice | | | | | | | ● |
| Papaya | ● | | | | | | |
| Peaches | ● | | | | | | |
| Peanut butter | | | | | | | ● |
| Pears | ● | | | | | | |
| Peas | | ● | | | | | |
| Quinoa | | | | | ● | | |
| Rice | ● | | | | | | |
| Spinach | | | ● | | | | |
| Squash | | ● | | | | | |
| Sweet potato | ● | | | | | | |
| Tofu | | | ● | | | | |
| Tomato | | | | | | | ● |
| Wheat | | | | | ● | | |
| Yogurt | | ● | | | | | |
| Zucchini | | ● | | | | | |

*This table contains information on suggested starting dates for various foods. Keep in mind that a baby should receive only one new food a week, and giving baby every food listed under each month is not recommended.

[1] Pureed berries can be offered gradually after 12 months. Whole berries still can cause gagging, so be careful to consider how well your child chews her food. Some berries cause diaper rash or skin rashes, so be aware.

[2] Uncooked honey has caused botulism and even death in children under age one. Do *not* feed infants uncooked honey before age one!

[3] In this book, *milk* refers to breast milk or formula until age one. Authorities differ on starting dates for whole milk—most suggest waiting until age one. For this reason, formula or breast milk is used in all the recipes for babies under age one. Follow the pediatrician's advice on when to start giving your child milk and watch closely for any allergic symptoms or reactions. Many infants just cannot tolerate milk too early, and it would be a shame to put their little bodies through misery by neglecting to notice signs of sensitivity to milk.

# Foods That Could Cause Problems

| Food | Problem | Do Not Give to Baby Before Age: |
|---|---|---|
| Apple pieces, whole grapes | Choking | 1 |
| Candy, cookies | Choking | 1 (Hold off as long as you can!) |
| Carrot sticks | Choking | 2 |
| Chocolate | Allergy, digestive problems, too much sugar | 3 (Hold off as long as you can. They don't need it!) |
| Egg whites | Allergy | 1 |
| Leafy vegetables | Gagging | 1½–2 |
| Milk | Allergy, intolerance | 1 |
| Peanut butter (not thinned) | Allergy, gagging | 2 |
| Popcorn | Choking | 2 |
| Uncooked honey | Botulism, and possibly death, can occur in babies under a year old. | 1 |
| Wheat | Allergy | 10–12 months |
| Whole berries | Allergy, digestive problems, choking | 1½–2 |
| Whole corn | Allergy, gagging, choking | 2 |
| Whole nuts or seeds | Allergy, choking | 3 |
| Whole raisins | Choking | 2 |

**Note:** This may be a good time to take a course in CPR and to learn how to deal with a baby or child who is choking.

# Chapter Seven

# Coping With Food Allergies

The thousands of additives found in some of our foods today make it increasingly difficult to pinpoint specific food allergies. It seems the more we learn about allergies, the more complex the subject becomes. The good news: Most children outgrow food allergies by the time they are toddlers. And more good news is that the Food Allergen Labeling and Consumer Protection Act of 2004 now requires food manufactured in the United States to clearly state on a product's label whether it contains these major food allergens: milk, egg, peanuts, tree nuts, fish, crustacean shellfish, soy, and wheat. This has been a huge help in avoiding the introduction of foods that could cause problems.

The Centers for Disease Control and Prevention estimates that less than 4% of children under 18 actually have a food allergy. However, their findings also reveal that from 1997-2007 the prevalence of reported food allergies increased 18% in that same age group. Statistics sometimes don't mean anything until you or someone you love becomes one. So, let's look at a few facts about food allergies and some ways to avoid or cope with them.

## Food allergies and/or food intolerance:
- Can occur at any age
- Can appear after eating a food that has never caused an allergic reaction before
- Can cause a reaction anywhere in the body

- Can cause symptoms to appear only after large amounts have been consumed
- Can cause symptoms to appear only when foods are eaten during a certain season of the year
- Can cause allergic reactions in one child in a family but not a sibling
- Do not cause the same reaction all the time
- Often occur in a variety of foods in the same food family

What a list! Now, how can this information be applied to avoid or identify potential food allergies? Let's look at a few definitions helpful in forming a better picture of what happens in the body when it is subjected to an allergic food substance. An *allergen* is defined as something that causes an allergic reaction. Food, dust, mold, pollens, and pets are common allergens. The body reacts to these allergens by producing antibodies, which help to neutralize the action of the allergen. A *food allergy* occurs when the body has an abnormal reaction after eating a particular food, causing one or more distressing symptoms to appear. Food allergies appear when allergens enter the body with a certain food and the body overproduces antibodies to counteract it. A food allergy causes an altered action, or intolerance, to take place in the body rather than a normal reaction.

*Food intolerances* trigger symptoms that are unpleasant but not as severe as an allergic response. These symptoms usually come on gradually. The most common is lactose intolerance. This occurs when the body can't digest the lactose (milk sugar) found in milk and dairy products. If the offending food can be avoided for a few months, sometimes the slow reintroduction of them at a later date will yield more favorable results.

## CAUSES OF ALLERGY

Authorities have several theories as to what causes an allergic reaction. Most research lists heredity as appearing to be the biggest factor in most food allergies. However, I must share a few words here about heredity and genetic conditions. You may or may not be drawn to the work of Bruce H. Lipton, PhD. He is an internationally respected cellular biologist whose cutting-edge research suggests that the power to control our lives is *not* genetically preprogrammed. His work strongly indicates this power originates from our minds. Lipton suggests that only about 5% of all "genetic" conditions are actually genetic—the rest are a result of environmental programming. You may want to explore this information and relate it to food allergies or other conditions. Lipton is the bestselling author of *The Biology of Belief,* as well as the recipient of the 2009 Goi Peace Award. You'll know if this information is calling to you so you can explore it further. Now, back to the overview of allergies.

Although it seems specific allergies are not transferred from parent to child, the tendency to react abnormally to various allergens *appears* to sometimes be transferred. Another possible cause of food allergy is overeating. Some bodies can only cope with a certain amount of an allergen; anything over this amount causes a reaction. There are doctors who believe certain stomach disturbances can cause food allergies.

What are the foods that can cause a food allergy? Any food can cause allergic reactions, but the most common foods are cow's milk, wheat, eggs, peanuts, tree nuts, soybeans, and crustacean shellfish. And for children, we need to add eggs to that list. Eggs are one of the most common allergy-causing foods in infants and children. Other foods that can cause problems are corn, citrus, seeds, and strawberries. Cinnamon, chocolate, and tomatoes also make the list of foods that frequently cause problems. Foods containing artificial additives and dyes are offenders as well.

The following foods are least likely to cause problems: rice, oats, barley, peaches, pears, bananas, applesauce, lettuce, carrots, grapes, squash, and sweet potatoes. If one or both parents have a tendency toward allergies, avoiding those foods might help to ensure baby gets an allergy-free start when solid foods are introduced in the diet.

Doris Rapp, MD, a well-respected board-certified environmental medical specialist, pediatric allergist, and homeopath, has written several books about allergies that are very helpful to the parent of an allergic child. *Is This Your Child* is an excellent resource.

## ALLERGY SYMPTOMS

Symptoms of allergy can range from minor (itchy skin or runny nose) to severe (convulsions or even death). Allergic symptoms can appear immediately after eating the offending food, or as long as several days afterward.

**The most common symptoms of food allergy are:**
Difficulty breathing
Itchy, runny nose
Swelling of lips or eyelids
Hives
Tightness of the throat
Wheezing
Headache
Asthma
Digestive problems (nausea, diarrhea, vomiting, gas)
Irritability
Fatigue
Behavior problems

## DEALING WITH FOOD REACTIONS

Should you suspect allergy but are not sure which food is the offender; try eliminating the foods most likely to cause allergy. An allergist with up-to-date training and experience with current methods of detecting allergies can be consulted to help discover specific food allergies.

If your child has a mild reaction to a given food, try waiting a few weeks before offering it again. If the same symptoms appear, eliminate that food from baby's diet. If baby has a violent reaction the first time a food is eaten, do not offer the food again. The risk is far too high. In rare instances, death has occurred as a result of a severe food allergy. If your baby has breathing difficulties or swelling of the tongue or throat, call 911. Baby will need immediate medical attention.

As you can see, food allergies are complex and not any fun for anyone involved. Prevention is a great strategy. If solid foods are introduced slowly, at not too early an age, and baby is given only one new food a week, parents have a better chance of preventing food allergies from occurring in their children.

The pages that follow include feeding information helpful for a child allergic to eggs, milk, wheat, or gluten. There is a Baby's Food Diary at the end of this chapter where you can record reactions to new foods.

You'll find recipes for a child with these particular allergies in chapter 13.

## EGG-FREE DIET

Eggs provide excellent nutrients, including protein, fat, and iron, but they are not an essential part of a diet. Watching out for foods containing eggs can be tricky, so label reading is a must.

Although recent advances in technology have reduced the risk of allergic reactions to childhood vaccines, it's important to know that some vaccines are still being cultured on eggs, causing allergic symptoms to appear in people who are extremely sensitive to eggs. Consult your child's doctor if you even suspect egg allergy in your child. Some people who are allergic to eggs are also allergic to chicken.

### Egg Substitutes

There are a few good substitutes for eggs when cooking or baking. A little bit of tofu can work quite well. Some recipes that call for one or two eggs can be replaced with a tablespoon or two of water. Baked goods are a little trickier. Mashed banana or applesauce can be substituted in many baked goods. Experimentation and imagination will be helpful here. People for the Ethical Treatment of Animals (PETA) offers these creative options to replace one egg: 1/4 cup pumpkin or squash, or 1/4 cup mashed potatoes, or 1/4 cup mashed pureed prunes.

The egg substitutes found in the supermarket are not always egg-free. Some of these are made for people concerned with low-cholesterol diet, so read the labels. Most natural food stores sell egg substitutes.

There is some optimistic news in desensitizing children with egg allergies. You may want to check out the July 2012 issue of the *New England Journal of Medicine* to learn more.

## Foods for Baby to Avoid on an Egg-Free Diet:

Beverages made with eggs: eggnog, malted shakes, root beer
Noodles or pasta made with eggs
Desserts made with eggs: ice cream, cookies, cakes, cream pies, meringue pies, custards, sherbets, candies
Hollandaise sauce, tartar sauce
Bread products made with eggs, breaded foods
Pancakes, waffles, French toast
Doughnuts
Pretzels
Dried or powdered eggs
Egg whites or yolks
Egg white solids
Egg albumen
Mayonnaise and salad dressings containing eggs
Meatloaf or meat dishes containing eggs
Cake mixes or other prepared mixes containing egg products or egg ingredients
Egg dishes (scrambled, baked, fried or boiled eggs, omelets, quiches, soufflés)
Poultry or fish dishes containing eggs
Baking powders that contain egg whites or albumen
Soups, any soup containing egg products or ingredients

## THE MILK-FREE DIET

Milk is one of the most common foods causing allergy. Waiting until after baby's first birthday to introduce milk seems to decrease the chance of an allergic response. And some suggest waiting until your child's second birthday to introduce milk. Whatever the starting date you choose, it does not guarantee that a milk allergy or intolerance will not occur. Symptoms of milk allergy can be mild or severe and include hives, wheezing, vomiting, and digestive problems. It's wise to be aware of any of these symptoms should they occur when milk is introduced, and stop feeding your child milk if symptoms appear. Avoiding milk products is the primary treatment for milk allergy.

There are two types of adverse reactions to milk: (1) lactose intolerance and (2) milk allergy. Some people have lactose intolerance, meaning their bodies have difficulty digesting milk. This is because they lack lactase, the enzyme responsible for the digestion of lactose (milk sugar). Symptoms of milk intolerance are abdominal cramps, bloating, diarrhea, and gas. Children (or adults) with milk intolerance can sometimes eat yogurt since the fermenting process involved has already broken down the milk sugar, making it easier to digest. Lactase can be purchased to add to whole milk (24 hours before using it) to make it more digestible for the intolerant person. For those who just can't do without milk, lactase-treated milk products are now available next to the regular milk at your grocery store.

A milk allergy is more severe than milk intolerance. People with a milk allergy must avoid all milk and milk products. Although cow's milk is the usual cause of milk allergy, other kinds of milk (sheep, goat, buffalo, and soy milk) can also cause a reaction. Yogurt or lactase-treated products would not benefit them since they are allergic to the milk itself. The good news is the Mayo Clinic reports that most children outgrow a milk allergy by age three.

Once it is known or suspected a child is allergic to milk, alternatives need to be found. The knowledge of which foods are necessary to avoid is very important.

## Foods for Baby to Avoid on a Milk-Free Diet:

All milk beverages: milk, milkshakes, cocoa, chocolate milk, half-and-half, condensed milk, evaporated milk, skim milk, 1% milk, 2% milk, powdered milk, dried milk, milk solids, curds and whey

Butter, margarine (check labels: some margarine is milk-free but it is also typically laden with artificial ingredients)

Cream, sour cream, whipping cream, buttermilk

Cheeses (including cottage cheese)

Yogurt

Custards

Breads, biscuits, muffins, pancakes, waffles, crackers made with milk or milk products
Cookies, cakes, ice cream, puddings, doughnuts, pies, desserts made with milk or milk products
Creamed soups, vegetables, sauces, gravies
Canned or dehydrated soups made with milk or milk products
Milk chocolate
Mashed potatoes (if milk has been added)
Salad dressings containing milk or milk products
Casein, sodium caseinate and lactalbumin (Watch closely for these particular milk proteins when reading labels. Some non-dairy products and some canned tuna fish contain casein. Some meats use casein as a binder.)

Once you know or suspect your child is allergic to milk, consult immediately with a health care provider who has knowledge and experience in dealing with milk allergies. She will suggest alternatives to meet your child's needs. Also ask your child's pediatrician to be sure there are no milk products, including whey, in any medications prescribed for your little one.

## WHEAT-FREE DIET

Wheat is another food that frequently causes allergic reactions. Rice, barley, and oats are usually the first cereals offered baby in order to avoid possible allergic reactions. (See information about oats in the gluten-free section, since oats can be contaminated with wheat during growing and processing.)

### Foods for Baby to Avoid on a Wheat-Free Diet:
Flour: white, whole wheat, enriched, unbleached, graham
Wheat bran or wheat germ
Wheat gluten or wheat starch
Malt, malted milk
Farina
Monosodium glutamate
Breads, biscuits, muffins, rolls, crackers, pretzels
Doughnuts

Pancakes, waffles
Breadcrumbs
Pasta
Desserts made with flour (pies, cakes, cookies, candies)
Gravy, sauces, tamari sauce
Processed cheese (some contain wheat stabilizers)
Some meat products (canned meats, hot dogs, sausage, meatloaf, lunch meats)

**Good substitutions for 1 cup of wheat flour:**
1¼ cups rye flour
1½ cups oat flour
⅝ cup potato flour
⅞ cup rice flour
¾ cup barley flour
¾ cup cornmeal

Experimentation and perseverance will be necessary when substituting other flours for wheat flour, since some recipes work better than others when substituting different types of flours.

## GLUTEN-FREE DIET

Gluten is a protein found primarily in wheat, barley, and rye. It is also found in variations or hybrids of those grains: spelt, triticale (a cross between wheat and rye), faro, and grano. Gluten is actually a protein complex containing gliadin and glutenin. When baking bread containing wheat flour, these two proteins combine to create gluten, which result in dough that traps gas bubbles created by the yeast, causing the dough to rise.

Oats can be gluten-free but they can also be contaminated with wheat during growing and processing. For this reason, the recommendation is to avoid oats unless they are specifically labeled gluten-free. And remember, just because it says gluten-free on the label, it doesn't mean those pretzels, cookies, or chicken-nuggets are healthy.

Speaking of labeling, as of this writing, the Food and Drug Administration (FDA) has still not approved a definition for "gluten-free" and has not taken the steps needed to create regulated standards for labeling. Several organizations provide independent certification: the Celiac Sprue Association, the Gluten Intolerance Group's Gluten-Free Certification Organization, and the National Foundation for Celiac Awareness currently certify products and companies as gluten-free. The National Foundation for Celiac Awareness recently partnered with Quality Assurance International and recommends their gluten-free product certification. Each program tests for different levels of gluten, with The Celiac Sprue Association appearing to be the strictest in its certification process.

When reading through the maze of labels, note that a certified gluten-free item will always be wheat-free but a wheat-free item may not always be gluten-free. Many grains, for example rice or oats, typically do not contain gluten but can be processed on equipment that could cause cross-contamination. Look closely at the labels if your child has these sensitivities or allergies.

Why is gluten a problem for some children and adults? It can cause inflammation in the small intestines resulting in gluten intolerance, or if it's more severe, it results in celiac disease. Babies with celiac disease or gluten intolerance may show these symptoms:

- Failure to thrive
- Loose stools, constipation, or both
- Bloating and gas
- Skin rashes
- Irritability
- Vomiting

Many healthy and delicious foods are naturally gluten-free including vegetables, fruits, beans, seeds, nuts (in their natural, unprocessed form), fresh eggs, fish (not breaded, coated, or marinated), and most dairy products.

Many grains and grain-like cereals or seeds can be part of a gluten-free diet. It's important to be sure they have not been processed with gluten-containing grains and that they do not have gluten additives or preservatives.

## Gluten-free grains include:

Amaranth
Buckwheat
Corn and cornmeal (non-GMO)
Flax
Millet
Oats (not grown near wheat fields and labeled "gluten-free")
Quinoa
Rice
Sorghum
Soy (non-GMO)
Teff

## Gluten-free flours include:

Almond
Amaranth
Arrowroot
Chia
Chickpea
Corn
Hemp
Millet
Potato
Quinoa
Rice
Sorghum
Soya
Teff

## Foods for Baby to Avoid on a Gluten-Free Diet:

Wheat (including bulgur, spelt, kamut, semolina, faro, and durum)
Barley (malt, malt flavoring, and malt vinegars are usually made from barley)
Rye
Triticale

# Baby's Food Diary

| Food Introduced | Baby's Age | Today's Date | Liked | Disliked | Adverse Reaction | Time Food Was Given | Time of Reaction |
|---|---|---|---|---|---|---|---|
| | | | | | | | |
| | | | | | | | |
| | | | | | | | |
| | | | | | | | |
| | | | | | | | |
| | | | | | | | |
| | | | | | | | |
| | | | | | | | |

# Chapter Eight

# BEGINNER RECIPES (SIX MONTHS)

The beginner recipes are for six-month-old babies who are starting to eat solid foods. Early feeding need not be elaborate and baby doesn't need a wide variety of choices. This section includes tips for introducing solid foods as well as recipes for making cereals and fruit purees. A slow introduction of each new food is recommended (see chapter 6).

Several timesaving ideas are included in this section:

- Making large batches of fruits to puree and freeze in ice cube trays
- Grinding grains ahead of time and storing in jars for daily use
- Using a pressure cooker
- Using the microwave safely

## INTRODUCING SOLIDS

Here are a few tips for those first days of introducing solid foods to your baby:

1. Choose a non-fussy time to begin feeding solid food. Between bottles or nursing is usually a good time.
2. Start with small spoonfuls of each new food. Feed gently and in a relaxed manner.

3. Never save foods that baby doesn't finish. The serving spoon mixes saliva into the remaining food and this saliva breaks down the food, causing a loss in nutritional value and freshness.
4. With the exception of bananas and avocados, fruits and vegetables should be cooked for babies until they are eight months old. They can digest them easier and there is less chance of choking.
5. Take time to enjoy baby's mealtimes. Household chores will always be there, but your infant won't stay little very long. Have fun!

## MICROWAVE SAFETY TIPS

I recommend stovetop cooking rather than using a microwave for any food, but you may make different decisions. Microwave ovens can be used for cooking large batches of vegetables and fruits. Cooking times vary with different models, foods, and amounts of foods. Check the manufacturer's instruction book to help guide you.

Always check the temperature of the food before giving it to baby. Reminder (in case you missed this in the previous chapters): Microwaves are not recommended for heating baby bottles since the liquid is heated unevenly and can cause severe and unexpected burns. Always use microwavable glass dishes since plastic containers may melt, releasing carcinogenic substances into baby's food.

## INTRODUCE (BEGINNING AT SIX MONTHS):

**Fruits**

applesauce
apricots
avocado
banana
papaya
pears
plums

Offer one new food a week, all in pureed form. One meal a day can be given for the first weeks of feeding solids. Gradually increase to two meals.

**Grains**
> barley
> millet
> oats
> rice

**Sample Menu for Beginners**
> Breakfast: Rice cereal
> Dinner: Apple puree
> Plus: Breast milk or formula

# AVOCADO-ADO

*2-3 tablespoons ripe, peeled avocado*

Mash with fork or blend with a baby food grinder. You can add breast milk or formula to make it thinner for the first few feedings.

A few words about the avocado: If you have never eaten an avocado, please don't toss this recipe aside. Avocados are a great first food for baby. They are soft, have a mild taste, and are rich in many nutrients. Please don't assume your baby won't like avocados if you have never tasted them—like I almost did! When choosing an avocado, purchase one that is soft (not mushy) to the touch, or buy a firm avocado and let it sit out a few days until it gets soft.

# BANANA-ANA

*½ ripe banana, peeled*

Mash with fork or blend with a baby food grinder. Add a bit of breast milk or formula to thin for initial feedings.

# AVOCADO BANANA CREAM
(Affectionately called "That Green Stuff")

*½ banana*
*¼-½ small avocado*

Blend thoroughly in a baby food grinder.


# FRUIT PUREE

*Large quantity of fruit (babies like apples, pears, blueberries, peaches, plums, goji berries, apricots) washed, peeled (except berries), and chopped*

Add *1/4* cup boiling water to each cup of fruit. Simmer until tender. Blend everything (including water) in blender. Freeze remainder in ice cube trays. Thaw 2 or 3 cubes when needed. Fruit can be served warm or at room temperature.

**Pressure cooker method:** Place washed, peeled whole fruit (remove seeds) on rack and add 1 cup water. Do not fill pressure cooker over two-thirds full. Cook according to the timetable below, allowing pressure regulator to rock slowly during cooking. Cool cooker under faucet of cool running water until pressure drops to normal or according to manufacturer's directions. Puree in blender or food processor and freeze in ice cube trays.

| Fruit | Cooking Time |
| --- | --- |
| apples | 7 minutes |
| apricots | 2 minutes |
| peaches | 5 minutes |
| pears | 6-8 minutes |
| plums | 2 minutes |

# DRIED FRUIT PUREE

*1 cup dried fruit (choose from apricots, blueberries, cranberries, papayas, peaches, pears, or apples). Add water to cover.*

Place in covered container and soak overnight in refrigerator. Pour into the blender the next day and puree. Serve and then refrigerate remainder no more than 3 days.

# DRIED FRUIT PUREE (Quick Method)

Pressure cooker method: Place dried fruit on rack and add water to cover. Do not fill pressure cooker over two-thirds full. Cook according to timetable below, allowing pressure regulator to rock slowly during cooking. Cool cooker under faucet of cool running water until pressure drops to normal. Puree in blender or food processor and freeze in ice cube trays.

| Dried Fruit | Cooking Time |
| --- | --- |
| apples | 6-8 minutes |
| apricots | 6-8 minutes |
| figs | 20-25 minutes |
| papaya | 8-10 minutes |
| peaches | 6-8 minutes |
| pears | 6-8 minutes |
| prunes | 6-8 minutes |

**Note:** Cooking time varies depending on fruit size, so use the longer cooking time for the larger-size fruits.

## RICE CEREAL

*1 cup water, breast milk or formula*
*¼ cup brown rice powder (brown rice ground in blender\*)*

In saucepan, bring liquid to boil. Sprinkle in rice powder, stirring constantly. Simmer covered for 10 minutes. This is good with pureed fruit. Serve warm.

\*To grind large amounts of rice, barley, millet or oatmeal, place 3/4 cup of grain in the blender and whiz at high speed, 20-30 seconds. Store in sterile glass jars. (Oatmeal can be ground in a food processor but the other grains do better in the blender.)

## BARLEY CEREAL

*1 cup breast milk, water, or formula*
*¼ cup ground barley (ground in the blender)*

Bring liquid to a boil. Add barley and simmer 10 minutes. Serve warm. (Add more liquid for thinner consistency.)

## OATMEAL

*¼ cup ground oats (don't use the instant kind—just grind regular oatmeal in blender or food processor)*
*¾ cup water*

Bring water to boil. Add oats, cover, and simmer 5 minutes. Serve warm with added breast milk or formula, or pureed apples or pears.

## RICE, OAT, OR BARLEY CEREAL
(Method 2)

Cook grains (without grinding them first) by regular method, omitting salt (see the Cooking Grains chart on page 124). After grains are cooked, blend in the blender or food processor until smooth. This is an easy way to cook cereal when other children or family members are eating the same foods together.

## MILLET CEREAL

*1 cup breast milk, water, or formula*
*3 tablespoons ground millet*

Bring liquid to a boil. Add millet, stirring constantly for a minute. Simmer 10 minutes. Serve warm.

## COMBINATION CEREAL

*¾-1 cup water*
*1 tablespoon ground oats*
*1 tablespoon ground rice*
*1 tablespoon ground barley*

Bring water to a boil. Add grains and stir with wire whip. Cover and simmer 10 minutes. Serve warm.

# Chapter Nine

# INTERMEDIATE RECIPES
# (SEVEN TO NINE MONTHS)

Intermediates (seven- to nine-month-olds) are getting the knack of being spoon-fed. Most of them are ready to venture into the world of vegetables and different cereal combinations. Introduced in this section are recipes for vegetables, cereals, yogurt, smoothies, tofu, and various lunch ideas. Baby should now be eating two meals a day and can enjoy a smoothie snack.

At this time, you may want to consider adding whole milk yogurt to your baby's menu. Babies will need the full-fat version with no added sugar or artificial sweetener. As mentioned in chapter 6, whole milk yogurt is usually tolerated very well at this age even though whole milk itself is not recommended for a baby before age one. The fermenting process of the milk breaks down the lactose (milk sugar) into lactic acid so that step in the digestive process is already completed by the time it reaches the stomach. Always be alert for possible milk allergy (symptoms may include hives, wheezing, or a rash) after introducing yogurt and other milk products. Milk intolerance can cause abdominal discomfort, bloating, diarrhea, and gas.

# INTRODUCE: (SEVEN TO NINE MONTHS)

**Mild vegetables**
    carrots
    green beans
    peas
    squash

**Yogurt**

**Egg yolks (cooked)**

**Beverages**
    fruit/veggie smoothies

**Tofu**

**Sample Menu for Intermediates**
    Breakfast: Oatmeal cereal plus apple puree
    Lunch: Tofu-banana whip or smoothie
    Dinner: Baby vegetable puree
    Plus: Breast milk or formula

> Continue introducing one new food per week. Begin combining fruits with cereals. Smoothies can be given for an occasional snack. Whole grain bagels or bread can be given to help with teething. Watch closely for choking or gagging. Gradually increase to three meals a day. Continue to puree most foods but begin to offer thicker, lumpier foods. Watch for food allergies.

# BABY VEGETABLE PUREE

*Large quantity of fresh vegetables (choose from carrots, green beans, peas, or squash)*

Add at least 2 inches of water in saucepan. Cover and cook until tender. Puree in blender (include the water in the blending); serve warm. Freeze remainder in ice cube trays.

**Pressure cooker method:** Using a pressure cooker to cook vegetables saves most of the valuable vitamins and minerals that can escape during regular cooking. Clean and chop vegetables; add 1/2 to 1 cup water and cook according to pressure cooker directions. Don't forget to include the cooking water when you puree vegetable in the blender. The pressure cooker method allows you to prepare a large quantity at a time.

## STEAMED VEGETABLES

*2 cups chopped fresh vegetables (choose from carrots, green beans, peas, or squash)*
*1½ cups water*

In a saucepan, bring water to a boil under the steamer basket. Wash vegetables and place in steamer basket. Check water level to be sure water is not touching vegetables. Cover and steam until tender (usually about 10 minutes if vegetables are cut small). Puree in blender along with cooking water. Serve warm. Freeze remainder in ice cube trays.

## CARROT & BEAN SOUP

*1 carrot, chopped*
*1 cup green beans, chopped*
*2 cups water*

Place all ingredients in a saucepan. Cover. Simmer until tender (about 30 minutes, depending on size of cut vegetables). Blend carrots, beans, and cooking water together in blender. Serve warm. For a larger batch, just increase all ingredients proportionately. Freeze remainder in ice cube trays for later use.

# HOMEMADE YOGURT

*4 cups whole milk*
*2 tablespoons whole plain yogurt or 1 package dried yogurt culture*

In a small bowl, add yogurt or culture to 1 cup milk and stir until dissolved. Pour into saucepan and then add remaining 3 cups milk. Mix well. Cook over low heat until milk starts to bubble around the edges of the saucepan. Remove from heat and cool to between 105°F and 115°F. (You'll need a cooking thermometer, or you can test the milk on your wrist. It should feel warm, not hot.) Remove 1 cup warm milk and place in a small bowl. Stir in yogurt or yogurt culture until dissolved. Add to remaining milk and stir again. Pour into individual containers of a yogurt maker or into sterile glass jars. Cover.

**Incubate in yogurt maker for 6 to 10 hours or use one of the following methods:**

- Place jars of yogurt on a heating pad and wrap tightly with towels or a small blanket.
- Place in electric oven on lowest possible temperature.
- Place a hot-water bottle at the bottom of a large cooking pot. Place yogurt on top and cover tightly. Wrap pan in towels.
- Place in metal cooking pan and place close to wood stove. (A constant temperature of 110°F is ideal during incubation period.)

**Helpful Yogurt-Making Tips**

- If using homemade yogurt for the culture, be sure it is used within five days.
- Do not use yogurt that contains stabilizers (or any additives). Read labels closely.
- Be gentle with yogurt. Fold gently when adding yogurt to other ingredients.
- Do not add fruit to yogurt during cooking time. Dried fruits should be added right before yogurt is put in the refrigerator. Other fruits should be added at serving time.

- Homemade yogurt tastes best if used within two weeks. After that time, yogurt is best used in cooking since it develops a sharper flavor.
- Yogurt can also be made with soy milk, brown rice milk, goat's milk, or oat milk. Wait to use almond milk until after age two due to possible nut allergy reactions.

## FRUIT YOGURT*

*3 tablespoons plain yogurt (full-fat)*
*2 tablespoons pureed fruit (apples, blueberries, peaches, bananas, or apricots)*

Mix together and serve. Most babies will love yogurt, even if their parents don't.
Note: The higher fat content in whole milk yogurt makes it easier to digest.

*No whole berries until age two.

## SMOOTHIES

*½ cup fruit (berries, peaches, papaya, bananas, or apricots)*
*½ cup milk (breast milk or formula before age one)*
*¼ cup plain whole milk yogurt\**
*¼ teaspoon vanilla extract*
*1 teaspoon blackstrap molasses (or honey after age one)*

Blend in blender. Serves baby plus one!

*Although yogurt is easily digested and usually well tolerated by infants, a child with an allergy to milk will have an allergic reaction to yogurt because it is a milk product. If any reaction occurs, stop all milk products and check with the pediatrician for suggestions on when to reintroduce milk into baby's diet.

## SIMPLE BANANA SMOOTHIE

*½ cup plain yogurt*
*½ banana*
*¼ teaspoon blackstrap molasses (or honey after age one)*

Blend all ingredients in a blender. Serve at once. One serving. (Double the recipe if you want enough for a thirsty toddler and a friend.)

## OATMEAL PLUS

*1¼ cups water*
*¼ cup oatmeal (rice or barley can also be used)*
*¼ cup chopped dates, raisins, blueberries, acai berries, goji berries, peaches, or apricots*

Bring water to a boil. Add remaining ingredients. Cover and simmer for 5 minutes. Puree in grinder or blender. Serve warm.

## TOFU-BANANA WHIP

(Often called "toe-food" around our house)

*½ banana*
*1 tablespoon tofu*

Mash with fork and stir until smooth. You could also simple put these two ingredients in a baby food grinder to blend.

**Note:** Tofu can be introduced after your baby is eight months old. Tofu is made from soybeans similar to the way cheese is made from milk. Store tofu in the refrigerator and keep it covered with water. If the water is changed daily (or almost every day) tofu will last up to seven days. If it doesn't smell fresh, don't use it. Draining tofu on a paper towel helps remove excess water before you combine it with other ingredients. Tofu is a good source of protein and is usually found in the produce department at your grocery store. Check the date to ensure freshness. Choose organic when you can.

## BABY RICE PUDDING

*½ cup brown rice*
*2 cups milk (formula, breast milk or water before age one)*
*1 egg yolk (or whole egg after age one)\**
*1 teaspoon blackstrap molasses*

Rinse rice. Combine all ingredients in saucepan. Bring to a boil, then simmer 1 hour. Check a few times to see if more liquid needs to be added. Let cool. Blend with blender or baby food grinder. Good served warm or cold.

*Reminder: Babies should not be given eggs whites before age one.

*Chapter Ten*

# ADVANCED RECIPES (TEN TO TWELVE MONTHS)

Advanced babies are getting more lovable by the minute. Many ten-, eleven- and twelve-month-olds are sprouting a few teeth, and their gums are all set for exploring lumpier foods. These babies begin to see a lot of options available on their menu. Grains, beans, cooked egg yolks, and a wider variety of vegetables are now menu options. You'll find two charts in this chapter that can serve as a guide to cooking various types of beans and grains. Be alert for wheat or egg allergies and be careful not to overfeed. Remember to let baby use her teeth and gums to chew or mix the food.

## INTRODUCE: (TEN TO TWELVE MONTHS)

**Legumes**
    cooked dried beans and peas

**Grains**
    bulgur
    quinoa
    wheat

Meals can begin to be in less pureed form but avoid large chunks of food. Finger foods can be offered. Continue to watch for reactions or allergies to any new (or old) food. Advanced-age babies can have three meals a day plus healthy snacks.

**Vegetables**
  broccoli
  kale
  cauliflower

**Cheese**
  cottage cheese
  small cheese cubes
  shredded melted cheese (warm, not hot)

**Sample Menu for Advanced Babies**
  Breakfast: Quinoa Delight with fruit puree
  Lunch: Lentils & Rice or Carrot-Zucchini Shred
  Dinner: Rice & Beans and mashed carrot or soft carrot pieces, or
  Garden Casserole and whole grain bread or rice crackers
  Plus: Breast milk or formula

# QUINOA DELIGHT

*1 cup whole quinoa*
*2 cups water*

Rinse quinoa. Combine quinoa and water in a saucepan. Cover and bring to boil. Reduce heat and simmer on low heat for 10 minutes. Add mashed banana for a change of pace.

# QUINOA & VEGETABLES

*¾ cup boiling water*
*⅓ cup quinoa (or bulgur)*
*2 tablespoons grated zucchini*
*2 tablespoons grated carrot*
*1 tablespoon shredded cheese (optional)*

If you are using quinoa, rinse it first. Bring water to a boil in a saucepan. Sprinkle quinoa (or bulgur), zucchini, and carrot into water and stir gently. Cover and simmer on low heat for 10 minutes. Blend through baby food grinder. Sprinkle with cheese and stir. Serve warm.

## LENTILS & RICE

¼ *cup cooked lentils*
¾ *cup cooked brown rice*

Blend together and puree with a little cooking water from the lentils. Serve warm. This makes 2 servings.

## RICE & BEANS

*3 tablespoons cooked brown rice*
*1 tablespoon cooked beans (pinto, black or other beans)*
*2 tablespoons cooking water from beans*
*1 tablespoon shredded cheese*

Mix all ingredients. Heat in a saucepan until cheese melts. Blend with grinder or serve as is if baby is receptive to lumpy food. This is an excellent protein dish.

## BROCCOLI & RICE

*1¼ cup chopped, cooked broccoli*
*½ cup cooked brown rice, rinsed quinoa, or bulgur*
*¼ cup cooked barley*
*¼ cup cooking water from broccoli*
*2 tablespoons grated cheese*

Combine first four ingredients and heat in a saucepan (no longer than 2-3 minutes since broccoli and grains are already cooked). Put through a baby food grinder and top with cheese or serve as is if your baby can chew lumpy food. This makes enough for two servings (one for dinner and one reheated the next day for lunch).

# Bean Preparation

| Use 1 Cup of | Soaking Required | Water | Cooking Time | Approx. Yield |
|---|---|---|---|---|
| **Baby Limas** Casseroles & side dishes | Yes | 2 cups | 1½ hrs. | 1¾ cups |
| **Black-eyed Peas** Main dishes & southern cookery | Yes | 3 cups | 1 hr. | 2 cups |
| **Black Beans** Soups & Mexican dishes | Yes | 4 cups | 1½ hrs. | 2 cups |
| **Garbanzos (chick peas)** Soups, salads, & dips | Yes | 4 cups | 2½-3 hrs. | 2 cups |
| **Great Northern Beans** Baked beans, soups, & main dishes | Yes | 3½ cups | 2 hrs. | 2 cups |
| **Kidney Beans** Chili & Mexican dishes | Yes | 3 cups | 1½-2 hrs. | 2 cups |
| **Lentils** Soups & casseroles | No | 3 cups | 1 hr. | 1 ¼ cups |

| Use 1 Cup of | Soaking Required | Water | Cooking Time | Approx. Yield |
|---|---|---|---|---|
| **Lima Beans** Side dishes & casseroles | Yes | 2 cups | 1½-2 hrs. | 1 ¼ cups |
| **Navy Beans (white beans)** Main dishes | Yes | 3 cups | 2½-3 hrs. | 2 cups |
| **Pea Beans** Baked beans | Yes | 3 cups | 2 hrs. | 2 cups |
| **Pinto Beans** Refried beans, chili, main dishes, & Mexican dishes | Yes | 3 cups | 2 hrs. | 2 cups |
| **Soybeans** Soups, main dishes, & casseroles | Yes | 4 cups | 3 hrs. | 2 cups |
| **Split Peas** Soups & main dishes | No | 3 cups | 1 hr. | 2 ¼ cups |

## How to Cook Beans

Rinse beans well under cold running water. Discard any cracked beans and small rocks while rinsing. Soak beans overnight. (Soybeans must be soaked in the refrigerator, but all other beans can remain at room temperature.) Place beans and water in a saucepan (use soaking water and add more water if necessary). Cover loosely and simmer for approximate amount of time specified above. Do not add salt or oil during cooking. A clove of garlic or small onion may be added if desired. Test beans for tenderness and adjust cooking time accordingly since the exact time varies.

## Quick soak method
Forget to soak the beans the night before? Bring water and beans to a boil. Simmer 2-3 minutes, then cover and let soak for 2 hours. Cook beans according to above directions.

## How to Cook Grains
Bring water to boil in a saucepan. Slowly sprinkle grain into boiling water. Cover and simmer over low heat for the amount of time specified in above chart. Do not add salt during cooking time.

# Cooking Grains

| Use 1 Cup of | Water | Cooking Time | Approx. Yield |
|---|---|---|---|
| Barley | 3 cups | 1hr., 15 min. | 3½ cups |
| Brown rice | 2 cups | 1 hr. | 3 cups |
| Buckwheat groats | 2 cups | 15 min. | 2 ½ cups |
| Quinoa (rinsed) | 2 cups | 5-10 min. | 4 cups |
| Bulgur wheat | 2 cups | 15-20 min | 2 ½ cups |
| Cracked wheat | 2 cups | 25 min. | 3 cups |
| Cornmeal | 4 cups | 25 min. | 3 cups |
| Millet | 3 cups | 45 min. | 3 ½ cups |
| Oatmeal | 2 cups | 15 min. | 2 cups |
| Whole wheat berries | 3 cups | 1 hr. | 2 ¼ cups |
| Wild rice | 3 cups | 1 hr. | 4 cups |
| Basmati rice | 1 cup | 20 min. | 2 ½ cups |

# RICE-SQUASH

*2 tablespoons squash (acorn, green, yellow)*
*2 tablespoons cooked brown rice*

Gently steam squash until tender. Pour into a small saucepan and stir in the cooked brown rice until the rice is warm. Blend in blender or grinder. This is good to have when rice is included in the family menu.

# COLORFUL BARLEY

*1 cup water*
*1 tablespoon uncooked barley, finely ground*
*1 tablespoon peas*
*½ carrot, grated*

Bring water to a boil. Sprinkle barley powder into the pan and stir with wire whisk or fork. Add peas and grated carrot. Simmer 15 minutes or until vegetables are tender. Serve warm.

# GARDEN CASSEROLE

*Broccoli*
*Cauliflower*
*Kale*
*Carrots*
*Potatoes*
*Cheese*

Chop vegetables and steam until tender. Top with a bit of baby's favorite cheese and serve warm.

## LENTIL CHEESEBURGERS

*½ cup lentils*
*1 egg yolk*
*1 tablespoon whole wheat bread crumbs or wheat germ*
*Dash of thyme (optional)*
*Monterey Jack or Swiss cheese slices (optional)*

Cook lentils until soft so they mash easily with a fork, about 1 hour. Drain any excess water and save for soup stock. When lentils are cool, add egg yolk, breadcrumbs, and thyme. Shape into patties. Bake 15 minutes at 350°F. Top with cheese slices and return to oven until cheese melts. Serve warm. (Be sure cheese has cooled to avoid a bad burn.)

## WHOLE WHEAT PANCAKES

*⅓-½ cup whole wheat flour*
*1 teaspoon baking powder*
*1½ teaspoons honey*
*½ cup milk*
*1 egg yolk or 1 tablespoon tofu*
*1½ teaspoons extra virgin olive oil*

Combine dry ingredients. Combine liquid ingredients. Stir into dry ingredients only until moistened. Cook in lightly oiled skillet. This makes enough for 2 servings. Refrigerate leftover pancakes for next day. Reheat briefly in dry skillet, just till warm. Serve with yogurt and fruit.

Note: Babies enjoy picking up bite-size pieces and feeding themselves.

## ZUCCHINI PANCAKES

*1 zucchini, grated*
*1 egg yolk (whole egg after age one)*
*2 tablespoons mashed tofu (optional—this can replace the egg)*

*½ cup whole wheat flour*
*⅓ cup milk*
*¼ teaspoon baking powder*

Mix all ingredients just until moistened. Cook in oiled skillet until lightly browned, just like regular pancakes. This is a great finger-food favorite. Save leftovers and reheat the next day. These also freeze well.

## SWEET POTATO PANCAKES

*2 sweet potatoes, finely shredded or processed in food processor*
*1 egg yolk (whole egg after age one) or 1 tablespoon tofu*
*2 tablespoons flour*

Combine all ingredients in mixing bowl. Pour batter by large spoonfuls onto oiled skillet. Flip when edges turn light brown. Serve at room temperature. This is another good finger food!

## APPLE DELIGHT

*½ apple, pared*
*½ banana*
*½ carrot*
*¼ cup water*

Blend in blender until smooth. This can be spoon fed to baby or served in a cup with larger holes in the lid. Apple Delight is a wonderful lunch served with rice crackers or toast.

## VEGETABLE LUNCH

*2 tablespoons zucchini, finely grated*
*2 tablespoons carrot, finely grated*

Blend in blender. Add yogurt for a different treat.

## CARROT SALAD

*7-8 presoaked raisins*
*2 tablespoons finely grated carrot*
*2 tablespoons finely grated apple*
*1 tablespoon yogurt*

Soak raisins in 1/2 cup water at breakfast, so they'll be soft by lunchtime. Be sure to blend raisins thoroughly in a blender or food grinder for children at this age. Wait until age one to introduce whole raisins. Some younger babies can handle them easily and others tend to gag a bit. Blend all ingredients through a baby food grinder and serve.

## COTTAGE CHEESE LUNCH

*Combine 3 tablespoons of cottage cheese with one of the following:*
*3 tablespoons applesauce*
*3 tablespoons pureed fruit*
*2 thawed fruit puree cubes (berries, apples, peaches, pears, apricots)*
*¼ small ripe avocado, mashed*

Blend in baby food grinder and serve.

## BUNNY YOGURT

*3 tablespoons carrot, finely grated*
*3 tablespoons yogurt*

Blend and serve.

# BUNNY YOGURT II

*2 tablespoons carrot, grated*
*2 tablespoons raw broccoli, grated*
*2-3 tablespoons plain yogurt*

Blend with a baby food grinder and serve. This makes a nice lunch served with whole grain toast and fruit pieces.

# CARROT-ZUCCHINI SALAD

*½ carrot, grated*
*½ zucchini, grated*

Steam carrot and zucchini in steamer 10 minutes or until soft. Blend in grinder with 2 tablespoons cooking water or serve as is to older baby. This can also be served raw after blending through processor or blender.

# BOILED SWEET POTATOES

Boil sweet potato (with the skin) for 30 minutes in a saucepan with water to cover the potato. Mash with a fork. Serve warm.

# BAKED ACORN SQUASH

*1 acorn squash*
*1 tablespoon honey*

Slice acorn squash in half. Scoop out seeds. Add honey to the center of each half. Bake on oiled pan at 350°F for 45 minutes or until tender. Greatly appreciated by adults, too!

## BABY'S FIRST BIRTHDAY CAKE

*2 cups whole wheat flour*
*½ teaspoon salt*
*2 teaspoons cinnamon*
*2 teaspoons baking soda*
*3 eggs*
*1½ cups canola or sunflower oil*
*¾ cup honey or brown rice syrup*
*2 cups carrots, grated*

Oil a 9" x 13" pan. Mix all dry ingredients and sift. Beat eggs, oil and honey; add to dry ingredients and mix. Fold in carrots. Bake 30 minutes at 350°F. Top with cream cheese icing.

## CREAM CHEESE ICING

*2 8-ounce packages cream cheese or Neufchatel cheese*
*¼ cup cooked honey*
*1 teaspoon vanilla*
*1 tablespoon butter (optional)*

Have cream cheese and butter at room temperature. Blend all ingredients.

Note: Cream cheese is high in saturated fat and not high on the list of cheeses that offer quality nutrients. It should be used sparingly or can be replaced with kefir cheese, yogurt cheese, Neufchatel cheese, tofu, or cottage cheese and whipped in the blender.

## GINGERBREAD SHORTCAKE

*½ cup butter*
*1 cup molasses*
*1 cup yogurt*

*2⅓ cups flour*
*Dash salt*
*¾ teaspoon baking soda*
*1 teaspoon cinnamon*
*1 teaspoon ground ginger*
*¼ teaspoon ground cloves*
*2 bananas, sliced*

Combine butter and molasses in a small saucepan and bring to a boil. Add yogurt. Sift all dry ingredients and add to molasses mixture and stir. Pour into square baking pan and bake at 350°F for 40 minutes. At serving time, remove from pan and cut into squares. Split squares into two layers and place sliced bananas between the layers. After age one, you can top the shortcake with a bit whipped cream. This is especially good served warm on a special occasion.

# Chapter Eleven

# TODDLE FOOD RECIPES (ONE TO THREE YEARS)

As baby begins to toddle about (at around age one), then run about (here come the terrific twos and threes), he needs especially nutritious foods available when he stops for a moment to grab a bite to eat. And often "a bite to eat" is all he'll settle for. He is too busy exploring his fascinating world. It seems at times as if two-year-olds live on air. Other times they'll attempt to clean out your refrigerator—with or without your help!

Nutritious finger foods are essential for toddlers. Here are a few foods they can grab on the run: fresh veggies, fruit pieces, cheese cubes, rice cakes, and rice crackers. When toddlers feel like having a real meal, they can be given many good foods from the whole family recipes. Various beverages (including water) and homemade Popsicles can provide essential vitamins and minerals between meals.

Along with a variety of recipes especially enjoyed by toddlers, I've included two recipes to help out mom or dad on a cold or rainy day. Laura's Play Dough and Kid's Stuff are two non-edible recipes to help make the day more enjoyable for all. Have fun during this wonderful, growing, and toddling time!

Milk in the recipes for children over the age of one can be cow's milk, goat's milk, soy milk, rice milk, oat milk, almond milk, or hemp milk. Enjoy making your own nut milks if you like and check labels if you are purchasing store-bought milks.

# INTRODUCE (ONE TO THREE YEARS):

Nutritious finger foods, new vegetables, fruits, or grains
Thinned peanut butter and other nut butters (be alert for nut allergy)
Nut milks and other milk sources: rice, soy, or hemp milk

> Three meals a day plus a snack or two can be given. Foods are lumpier and rarely need to be blended in the baby food grinder. Be sure all snacks are healthy ones since toddlers do not always stop to eat a complete meal. Continue to watch closely for signs of allergies.

### Sample Menu for Toddlers

Breakfast: Granola or muesli with milk or yogurt, and fruit
Snack: Veggies or fruit pieces
Lunch: Broccoli, quinoa, carrot pieces
Snack: Molly's Juice Bar, blueberries, vegetable pieces, or a smoothie
Dinner: Whole Wheat Pizza and salad or Falafel Burgers in pita bread, served with green beans
Plus: Breast milk or 2-3 servings of milk (cow, goat, nut, rice, soy, or hemp milk)

# ALMOND MILK

*1 cup raw organic almonds plus filtered water to cover during soaking*
*4 cups filtered water*
*Optional: vanilla bean, honey, or stevia*

Soak almonds overnight in the refrigerator. The next day, drain the water and put almonds in the blender. Add the 4 cups of water and blend on high speed for about 2 minutes. Pour almond mixture through a cheesecloth, strainer, or nut milk bag. Add a vanilla bean or a bit of honey or stevia if you like. Squeeze to get all the liquid you can. Store the almond milk in the fridge for up to 3 days.

# HEMP MILK

*1 cup shelled hemp seeds*
*6 cups filtered water*
*A bit of stevia to sweeten*

Blend hemp seeds and water in a blender on high for 2 minutes or in a Vitamix for 1 minute. Pour through cheesecloth or a nut milk bag then stir in the stevia. You can compost the remaining pulp.
Makes 6-7 cups and keeps well in the refrigerator for 3 days.

# NUT MILK

Use a blender to liquefy 2 ounces (1/3 to 1/2 cup) of sesame seeds, raw cashews, or blanched almonds with 6 ounces (3/4 cup) of water. This is good for making "milk" shakes for those not sensitive to these seeds or nuts.

# SOY MILK

Blend 1/4 cup tofu with 2/3 cup water in blender. Soy milk can be used for beverages or in baking.

# NUT BUTTERS

(A peanut butter substitute for people who are allergic to peanuts)

*1 cup ground nuts or seeds (almonds, sunflower seeds, or sesame seeds)*
*1 tablespoon sunflower or olive oil*

Lightly toast ground nuts or seeds in 300°F oven. Stir often. Place 1/4 cup ground nut meal in the blender with a small amount of oil. Blend at high speed for 5 seconds. Gradually add remaining nut meal (1/4 cup at a time) and oil and continue to blend. Stir mixture before each addition of nuts (be sure blender is turned off). Store nut butter in a glass jar in refrigerator. Use as peanut butter substitute or as a delightful addition to the diet.

Note: Some people who are allergic to peanuts may also be allergic to other nuts. So watch for allergic reactions.

## SUNNY SMOOTHIE

*¼ cup yogurt or milk (coconut milk is a great choice)*
*¼ cup orange juice (fresh-squeezed is preferred)*
*½ banana*
*¼ teaspoon blackstrap molasses or 1 teaspoon honey*
*Dash of vanilla extract*

Blend all ingredients in blender. Serve at once. A great dessert treat! Serves 1.

## CAROB MILK

*1 cup milk*
*1 tablespoon melted carob chips or 1 tablespoon carob powder*
*2 teaspoons honey*

Blend in blender and drink. Serves 1.

## CAROB DELIGHT

*1 cup milk*
*2 teaspoons carob powder*
*2 teaspoons honey*
*1 teaspoon non-instant dry milk*
*¼ teaspoon lecithin granules (optional)*

Blend all ingredients in the blender. Serves 1.

## PEGGY'S KALE SMOOTHIE

*1 apple, cut and cored*
*1 large or 2 small kale leaves (stems removed)*

*½ lemon, juiced*
*1 cup water (more if needed)*
*1 tablespoon honey*
*¼ teaspoon cayenne (optional)*

Blend and enjoy. Serves 1.

## AURORA'S ALMOND SMOOTHIE

*1 cup almond milk*
*1 banana*
*Handful of frozen cherries*

Blend and enjoy. You can also add a teaspoon of carob or cacao powder for a chocolate taste. Serves 1.

## BROWN MONKEY SHAKE

*1 cup milk*
*1 banana*
*2 teaspoons carob powder*
*1 teaspoon honey*
*1 teaspoon non-instant dry milk*

Blend in blender. Serves 1.

## BRONWYN'S SMOOSHIE

*1 cup of crushed ice*
*1 banana*
*4 strawberries*

Pour ice into blender and add banana and strawberries. Blend all ingredients in the blender until "smooshed." Serves 1 thirsty toddler. (I've heard this drink is also a favorite with teens.)

# GRANOLA

*4 cups old-fashioned oats*
*1 cup sesame seeds*
*1 cup sunflower seeds*
*1 cup wheat germ (raw)*
*1 cup unsweetened coconut*
*½ cup non-instant dry milk*
*½ cup honey*
*½ cup canola oil*
*1 teaspoon vanilla*
*½ cup almonds, chopped*
*½ cup raisins*

Toss dry ingredients (except raisins and almonds) in a large bowl. Mix honey, oil, and vanilla together and pour over oatmeal mixture; stir. Pour onto baking sheet and bake in 300°F oven for 30 minutes, stirring several times. Add almonds and raisins during the last 5 minutes. Remove from oven and cool completely before storing in a large glass jar with a tight-fitting lid.

# CORNMEAL CEREAL

*1 cup water*
*¼ cup yellow cornmeal*
*Dash of honey*
*A bit of milk to thin if necessary*

Using a double boiler, bring water to a boil. Slowly sprinkle cornmeal into water, stirring constantly with a wire whisk or wooden spoon. Simmer 15 minutes. Remove from stove and let stand 15 minutes. Add a dash of honey and thin with milk. Serves 1 toddler.

# BEAR MUSH DELUXE

Cook one serving of Bear Mush (Arrowhead Mills packaged cereal). Add 1 tablespoon of honey and 1/4 cup of chopped fruit (peaches, apricots, pears, or apples), and you have a delicious warm cereal on a cold winter morning!

## FRENCH TOAST

*1 egg*
*2 tablespoons milk*
*2 slices whole wheat bread*

Beat egg and milk together in a pie pan. Dip bread in egg mixture and place in oiled skillet. Cook on medium heat until lightly browned on each side. Good served with honey butter and cinnamon, or your favorite fruit preserves.

## HONEY BUTTER

*½ cup butter*
*½ cup honey*

Let butter soften at room temperature. Stir in honey with a fork. This is a great topping for waffles, pancakes, or French toast. Refrigerate after use.

## MEREDITH'S OMELET

*1 egg*
*1 tablespoon milk*
*½ teaspoon butter*
*2 tablespoons grated cheese*

Combine egg and milk and beat with a fork. Melt butter over low heat in a 7-inch skillet. Pour egg mixture into skillet and tilt skillet often so egg mixture becomes firm. Gently use a fork or wooden spoon to lift batter in some places so mixture touches hot skillet. When egg is cooked, add cheese and fold omelet in half. Keep in the skillet for 15 or more seconds; serve warm. Be sure that cheese has cooled enough for baby to eat safely. Green pepper, zucchini, or shredded cooked potato can also be added for variation.

Note: Be sure egg mixture is entirely cooked. Also, be on the lookout for allergic reactions to eggs.

## PITA-PINTO SANDWICH

*½ cup cooked pinto beans, mashed (garbanzos or soybeans can also be used)*
*Pita bread*
*Tomato slices*
*Avocado slices*
*Shredded cheese (optional)*

Spread the beans into the pita bread; add tomato, avocado, and cheese. Serve as is or put under broiler for 5 minutes. Be sure cheese is cooled to avoid burns.

## PEANUT BUTTER DELIGHT

*½ banana, mashed*
*2 tablespoons peanut butter*
*2 tablespoons tofu*

Blend in baby food grinder and serve. Thin with breast milk or formula, if necessary. This is good on rice cakes, gluten-free crackers, or whole grain toast.

## ELIZABETH'S PEANUT BUTTER PUDDING

*2 tablespoons peanut butter*
*2 tablespoons applesauce or pureed apple*
*½ banana*

Blend with a baby food grinder or mash with fork. Serve at room temperature.

## PEANUT BUTTER DELUXE SANDWICH

*Peanut butter*
*Applesauce*
*Raisins (presoaked for toddlers under age two)*
*Crushed sunflower seeds*

Mix all ingredients together and spread on whole grain bread.

## FLYNN'S FAVORITE BAGEL

*Bagel*
*Monterey Jack cheese*

Top bagel with Monterey Jack cheese slices (and nothing else) and place in toaster oven until cheese melts. (Check to be sure cheese is cooled enough to eat.) Serve with orange slices.

## QUINOA, SQUASH, & APPLES

*1 cup cooked quinoa*
*Soft cooked apples, diced*
*Soft cooked yellow squash, diced*

Combine and serve.

## CHEESE TORTILLAS

*1 corn tortilla, buttered*
*Ricotta cheese or tofu*
*Grated Monterey Jack cheese*
*Sliced tomato*

Place lightly buttered corn tortilla under the broiler for 2 minutes. Remove. Spread tortilla with ricotta or tofu, then tomato slices, and top with the cheese. Broil until cheese melts. Cool to room temperature.

## COTTAGE CHEESE DELIGHT

¼ *cup cottage cheese*
¼ *cup pureed fruit (apples, pears, apricots, etc.)*
*1 tablespoons fresh-squeezed juice from an orange*

Blend together and serve. This is a real favorite!

## APPLESAUCE & RAISINS

½ *cup applesauce*
*8 presoaked raisins*

Blend in baby food grinder and serve.

## CHICKIE DIP

½ *cup water*
*1 cup cooked garbanzos (chickpeas), mashed*
⅓ *cup canola oil*
*3 tablespoons sesame seeds*
½ *teaspoon sea salt*
*1 clove garlic, crushed*
*3 tablespoons lemon juice*

Blend in blender or food processor. This delicious chickpea dip is great with veggies, crackers, or as a sandwich spread.

## TODDLE SALAD

*1 apple*
*8 presoaked raisins*

*2 tablespoons shredded carrot*
*3 tablespoons yogurt*
*1 teaspoon honey or brown rice syrup*

Cut apple into bite-size pieces. Mix with raisins that have soaked overnight. Add carrot. Mix yogurt and honey and pour over salad. Serves 1.

## LENTIL STEW

*1 tablespoon celery, chopped*
*½ potato, cubed*
*½ carrot, grated*
*1 tablespoon oil*
*¼ cup washed lentils*
*1¼ cups water or vegetable broth*
*1 tomato, chopped, or ½ cup tomato juice*

Sauté celery, potato, and carrot in oil over medium heat. Add lentils, water, and tomato. Bring to a boil. Cover and simmer 1 hour. Stir on occasion. Add more water if needed.

## WHOLE WHEAT BISCUITS

*2 cups whole wheat flour*
*2 tablespoons bran*
*1 tablespoon baking powder*
*¼ cup non-instant dry milk*
*½ teaspoon salt*
*⅓ cup safflower oil*
*¾ cup milk*

Gently combine dry ingredients with wet ingredients. Knead 1 minute. Roll on floured cloth until 1/2-inch thick. Cut with biscuit cutter (star shapes or heart shapes are fun) and place on baking sheet. Bake at 450°F for 10 minutes. Makes 1 dozen.

## CORN MUFFINS

*1 cup cornmeal*
*¼ cup whole wheat flour*
*3 tablespoons soy flour (can be replaced with whole wheat flour, but the soy flour adds extra protein)*
*2 teaspoons baking powder*
*1 teaspoon salt*
*1 egg*
*1 cup milk*
*3 tablespoons non-instant dry milk*
*3 tablespoons honey*
*3 tablespoons oil*

Combine dry ingredients. Mix together all liquid ingredients. Add liquid mixture to dry ingredients and beat well. Bake in muffin cups or well-oiled muffin tin at 375°F for 20 minutes.

## PEANUT BUTTER BREAD

*2½ cups whole wheat flour*
*1 tablespoon baking powder*
*1 teaspoon salt*
*1¼ cups milk*
*¼ cup honey*
*2 tablespoons oil*
*¾ cup peanut butter*

Mix dry ingredients together. Set aside. Heat milk until warm. Add honey, oil, and peanut butter to milk and stir well. Add liquid mixture to dry ingredients and blend well. Pour into well-oiled bread pan and bake at 350°F for 40-50 minutes. This is delicious served with mashed banana.

## RAISIN AND BRAN MUFFINS

*3 cups bran*
*1 cup boiling water*
*2 eggs*
*1 cup honey*
*½ cup safflower oil*
*2 cups buttermilk*
*2¼ cups whole wheat flour*
*2 teaspoons baking soda*
*½ teaspoon sea salt*
*½ cup raisins*

Mix bran and boiling water in a large bowl and set aside. In another bowl, mix the eggs, honey, oil, and buttermilk. Add to the bran mixture. Sift together flour, baking soda, and salt and stir into bran mixture. Add raisins. Bake at 375°F in muffin tins (oiled or papered) for 15 minutes. Serve with butter or honey. Makes 2 dozen.

## OATMEAL MUFFINS

*2 cups oats*
*1½ cups buttermilk*
*1 cup whole wheat flour*
*1 teaspoon baking soda*
*½ teaspoon salt*
*2 eggs, beaten*
*3 tablespoons honey*

Mix oats with buttermilk. Set aside. Sift dry ingredients together and add to oat mixture. Stir in eggs and honey. Let mixture stand 20 minutes before baking. Bake at 375°F for 15-20 minutes in oiled or papered muffin tin. Makes 1 dozen.

# MICHAEL'S CORN TORTILLAS

*1½ cups water*
*3 tablespoons butter*
*1 cup cornmeal*
*1 teaspoon salt*
*1 cup whole wheat flour*

In a saucepan, bring water to a boil. Add butter. Stir in cornmeal and cook over low heat for 5 minutes. Cool. Add salt to the flour and combine with cornmeal mixture. (Add more water or flour if necessary.) Divide dough into 10-12 pieces. Roll out on floured board or pastry cloth into flat circles. Cook on a hot griddle or skillet 1½-2 minutes each side. Watch closely so they do not burn. Stack on a large plate and keep covered with a cloth. These are delicious topped with your favorite beans or cheese.

# FROZEN BANANAS

*Banana*
*Orange juice*

Insert a Popsicle stick in the banana (or in half a large banana). Dip in orange juice. Wrap in plastic wrap and freeze.

# MOLLY'S JUICE BARS

Pour diluted (50% water, 50% juice) from apples, oranges, grapes, apricots, or papayas into molds or cups with Popsicle sticks. These are good for teething babies but are sometimes difficult for them to hold alone. (You'll often find teething babies gnawing on the handles.)

# YOGURT POPSICLES

*2 cups plain yogurt*
*1 6-ounce can concentrated, unsweetened fruit juice (orange, apricot, grape, apple)*

*1 teaspoon vanilla extract*

Mix well and freeze in Popsicle molds or small paper cups with Popsicle sticks. These Popsicles are also great for teething babies.

## BANANA CRUNCHSICLES

*1 banana*
*2 tablespoons melted carob chips*
*½ teaspoon safflower oil*
*1 teaspoon honey*
*¼ cup granola*

Insert a Popsicle stick in one end of the banana. Mix carob chips, oil and honey together and melt over double boiler or in an egg poacher. Roll banana in melted carob mixture; then roll in granola. Freeze for several hours. Delicious!

## SPECIAL DAY SUNDAE

*1 scoop frozen yogurt*
*1 banana, sliced*
*½ cup fresh strawberries, sliced*
*1 tablespoon carob chips*
*Whipped cream*

Scoop yogurt into a dish. Cover with banana slices, strawberries, and carob chips. Top with a little fresh whipped cream.

## PEANUT BUTTER & OATMEAL COOKIES

*½ cup peanut butter*
*⅓ to ½ cup honey*
*1¼ cups old-fashioned oats*
*2 tablespoons dry milk*
*¼ teaspoon salt*

*¼ cup sunflower seeds (optional)*

Mix peanut butter with honey. Add dry ingredients and mix. Drop by rounded teaspoonfuls on oiled baking sheet. Bake 10 minutes at 350°F. Makes 2½-3 dozen.

## OATMEAL COOKIES

*1¾ cups flour*
*1 teaspoon sea salt*
*2 teaspoons baking powder*
*½ teaspoon cinnamon*
*⅓ cup safflower oil or softened butter*
*⅓ cup honey*
*⅓ cup molasses*
*2 eggs, beaten*
*2 cups old-fashioned oats*
*¾ cup raisins*

Sift together flour, salt, baking powder, and cinnamon. Combine oil, honey, molasses, and eggs in another large bowl. Add dry ingredients and mix well. Add oats and mix again. Gently stir in raisins. Drop by rounded teaspoonfuls on oiled cookie sheet. Bake at 350°F for 10-12 minutes. Makes 4 dozen.

## LAURA'S PLAY DOUGH

This is *not* to eat—but great for a rainy day project or a homemade birthday gift that children love.

*1 cup white flour*
*½ cup salt*
*2 tablespoons cream of tartar*
*1 tablespoon oil*
*1 cup water*
*Few drops food coloring (or juice from beets or blueberries)*

Mix flour, salt, cream of tartar, and oil in a saucepan. Add water and mix well. Cook over medium heat, stirring constantly, for 3 minutes. Dough will become difficult to stir and turn into clumps. Cool slightly and knead for 5 minutes. Add food coloring or juice during kneading process. This keeps a long time if stored in a tightly covered plastic container.

## KID'S STUFF

This recipe is *not* to eat—but another rainy day activity for toddlers and caregivers to enjoy. Holiday ornaments can be crafted or any old shape can be cut with cookie cutters.

*3 cups flour*
*1½ cups cornstarch*
*1 tablespoon dry mustard or instant coffee*
*1 cup water*

Combine dry ingredients in a large bowl. Pour in water, stirring constantly. Roll out on floured cloth or board and use cookie cutter for desired shapes, or shape and mold into shapes without cutting dough. Air-dry molded objects or bake 1 hour at 350°F. For a darker finish, brush first with milk and egg. Varnish when dry.

*Chapter Twelve*

# WHOLE FAMILY RECIPES

This chapter contains recipes for the entire family, ages 3 to 103! Many of these recipes can also be shared with a toddling two, but check ingredients closely to be sure the recipe does not contain any Foods That Could Cause Problems (see chart on page 91).

## BERRY GOOD OATMEAL

*1 cup old-fashioned oats*
*2 cups water*
*¼ cup blueberries, acai berries, or goji berries*
*½ cup chopped apples*

Bring water to boil. Sprinkle oats into water while stirring constantly. Cover and simmer 15-20 minutes on low heat. Remove from heat. Add berries and chopped apples. Cook 2 more minutes. Serves 2.

## SPECIAL DAY CEREAL

*1 scoop frozen yogurt*
*¾ cup granola or muesli*
*½ cup fruit (peaches, berries, bananas, strawberries)*
*¼ cup milk or yogurt*

Put yogurt in cereal bowl. Cover with granola or muesli, fruit, and milk. Enjoy!

## BAKED APPLE PANCAKE

*1 tablespoon oil*
*3 cups apples; sliced, peeled and cored*
*½ teaspoon cinnamon*
*½ teaspoon allspice*
*Juice from ½ lemon*
*½ cup whole wheat flour*
*¾ teaspoon baking powder*
*¼ cup honey*
*¼ cup yogurt or crumbled tofu*
*2 eggs*

Preheat oven to 400°F. Heat oil on low heat in a large saucepan or skillet. Pour in the apples, cinnamon, allspice, and lemon juice. Mix gently and then cover pan. Turn heat to medium and bring to a boil. Turn heat to low, cover, and simmer for 10 minutes. Remove from heat. Combine the flour and baking powder in a small mixing bowl. Pour in the honey, yogurt or tofu, and eggs. Mix with a fork just until smooth, about 30 seconds. Oil a 9-inch pie pan. Put about one-third of the batter in the bottom of the pie pan and spread around the bottom. Bake for 5 minutes. Remove from oven. Pour the apple mixture over the baked batter. Spoon the remaining batter over the apples and spread evenly, making sure the batter touches the edges of the pan. Bake 20-25 minutes. Cut in wedges. Serve warm.

## FAMILY WHOLE WHEAT PANCAKES

*¾ cup whole wheat flour*
*2 teaspoons baking powder*
*½ teaspoon salt*
*1 tablespoon honey*
*1 cup milk (whole milk or almond milk)*
*1 tablespoon oil*
*1 egg, beaten or 1 tablespoon mashed tofu*
*Berries or fruit preserves of your choice to top*

Mix the dry ingredients together in one bowl and the liquid ingredients in another. Add milk mixture to flour mixture and stir just until moistened (any lumps will disappear during cooking). Pour by spoonfuls into oiled skillet over medium heat. Flip when bubbles come to the top. These are ready when a golden color appears. Top with fruit or preserves.

## SUNFLOWER BREAD

*2 tablespoons oil*
*1 cup maple syrup or brown rice syrup*
*1 egg*
*¾ cup fresh-squeezed orange juice*
*2 tablespoons grated orange rind*
*1 tablespoon baking powder*
*½ teaspoon salt*
*2 cups whole wheat flour*
*1 cup sunflower seeds, raw or toasted*

Preheat oven to 325°F. Beat oil, maple syrup or rice syrup, and egg with electric mixer for 1 minute in a medium bowl. Combine remaining ingredients in a small bowl and add to first mixture all at once. Mix well with a wooden spoon just until smooth. Pour into oiled loaf pan and bake for 1 hour. Let cool in pan on rack 10-15 minutes. Turn out on rack to finish cooling. Wrap tightly to store.

## WHOLE WHEAT BREAD

*1 tablespoon dry yeast*
*2½ cups warm water*
*3 tablespoons honey*
*3 tablespoons olive oil*
*2 teaspoons sea salt*
*6 cups whole wheat flour*

Dissolve yeast in water with 1 tablespoon of the honey. When bubbles rise to surface (2-3 minutes), add remaining 2 tablespoons honey and oil. Combine salt and flour and add to mixture, about 1 cup at a time, using a wooden spoon for stirring. Knead for 10 minutes. Cover and let rise till double in bulk. Punch down, then separate into two oiled loaf pans. Cover and let rise again for 1 hour. Bake 30 minutes at 350°F.

## AVOCADO & ARUGULA SANDWICH

*Whole wheat or sunflower bread (or choose to wrap in a piece of washed Romaine lettuce)*
*1 tablespoon hummus*
*Avocado slices*
*Tomato slices*
*Romaine or arugula*
*Grated carrot*
*Cheese slices (optional)*

Toast the bread and spread with hummus. Add the avocado, tomato, grated carrot, and cheese. Cut in half and serve.

To serve a toddler, make this an open-face sandwich on one piece of toast and cut into fourths. Depending upon the age of the child, a lot of the sandwich will fall off. If this frustrates your child, you might try mashing up the avocado, bits of tomato, and grated carrot to make a sandwich spread to put on the toast. Variation: instead of toast, wrap ingredients in a large lettuce leaf.

## GREEK PITA SANDWICH

*Red or green peppers, sliced*
*Kale, chopped or in pieces*
*Onion, sliced*
*Tomato, sliced*
*Mushrooms, sliced*
*Goat cheese, feta cheese, or tofu, crumbled*

Cut a piece of pita bread so you have two flat pizza-like circles. Top each half with the vegetables and cheese or tofu. Pop into a broiler till cheese melts.

## EGG SALAD SANDWICH

*2 hard-boiled eggs, chopped*
*1 tablespoon celery, chopped*
*1 tablespoon onion, chopped*
*1 tablespoon safflower mayonnaise*
*Dash sea salt or Himalayan salt*
*Slice of your favorite healthy cheese*
*Handful of arugula*
*Pita bread, toasted bread, or bagel*

Combine egg, celery, and onion in a small bowl with enough mayonnaise to bind together. Add salt, to taste. Spread onto pita bread, toast, or a bagel. Top with a slice of cheese and a bit of arugula. Fresh tomato slices are also good.

## CHICK PEA DELIGHT

*2 cups cooked garbanzo beans*
*1 small clove garlic, crushed*
*2 tablespoons chopped green onion*
*2 tablespoons chopped red or green pepper or 2 tablespoons chopped celery or both*
*6 ounces tofu, drained*
*2 tablespoons soy sauce or 1 tablespoon tamari sauce*
*3 tablespoons safflower mayonnaise*

Mash garbanzo beans with a fork or quickly blend in blender or food processor. Add remaining ingredients and mix thoroughly. This spread is delicious on whole grain toast or rice crackers. You can add tomato, lettuce, or kale. It is also good served in whole wheat or gluten-free pita bread.

## RAINBOW SALAD

*Arugula, kale, chard, spinach and other favorite greens*
*Yellow pepper, cut into thin strips*
*Purple onion, chopped or sliced*
*Carrot, grated or sliced*
*Sugar snap peas*
*Broccoli (bite-size pieces)*
*Avocado (bite-size pieces)*
*Tomatoes, chopped*
*Daikon radish, sliced*
*Roasted pumpkin or sunflower seeds (to sprinkle on top)*

### Dressing:
*½ cup olive oil*
*½ cup lemon juice*
*Salt and pepper, to taste*
*Clove of garlic, crushed (optional)*

Wash salad greens and use a salad spinner or paper towel to gently dry leaves. Tear into bite-size piece and place in salad bowl. Chop or slice your choice of colorful raw vegetables and sprinkle all over the top. In a separate bowl, combine oil, lemon juice, salt, pepper, and garlic. Gently drizzle over the salad and toss. Sprinkle the top with the roasted seeds. Enjoy!

## FRUIT SALAD

*Grapes*
*Bananas*
*Oranges*
*Apples*
*Pineapple*
*Raisins*
*Coconut Melon*
*Watermelon*
*Pears*

Wash fruit and chop into bite-size pieces. Toss all fruit together in a large bowl and serve.

## SESAME SEED SALAD DRESSING

*¼ cup honey*
*½ teaspoon paprika*
*½ teaspoon salt*
*¼ teaspoon dry mustard*
*1 teaspoon onion juice or finely grated onion*
*½ teaspoon organic Worcestershire sauce*
*1 cup oil*
*½ cup cider vinegar*
*1 tablespoon toasted sesame seeds*

Blend all ingredients except sesame seeds in blender. Add seeds and mix with a spoon. This is a great "sweet and sour" dressing—especially good on spinach salads and falafel.

## TABOULI

*1½ cups bulgur wheat*
*¾ cup hot water*
*3 green onions, chopped*
*2 carrots, chopped*
*2 stalks celery, chopped*
*2 large tomatoes, chopped*
*⅓ cup olive oil*
*1¼ cup lemon juice*
*½ teaspoon sea salt*
*2 tablespoons chopped mint (optional)*
*2 tablespoons chopped parsley or cilantro (optional)*

Place bulgur in a large bowl. Add hot water, cover, and let stand while vegetables are being chopped. Prepare vegetables and add to the bulgur. Mix oil, lemon juice, salt, and herbs together and pour over the bulgur mixture. Chill at least 1 hour. Serve chilled.

Note: You can use 1½ cup cooked quinoa instead of bulgur. No need to add the hot water since the quinoa is cooked. Just add the vegetables, oil, lemon juice, salt, and your choice of fresh herbs. Chill and enjoy.

## SPINACH SALAD

*Spinach pieces, washed and dried*
*Mushrooms, sliced*
*Green onions, chopped*
*Hard-boiled egg, sliced (optional)*
*Provolone cheese, grated*

Toss all ingredients with Sesame Seed Salad Dressing and serve. A toddler might like a plate with all these ingredients separated. The cheese could be cubed instead of grated.

## ANTIPASTO SALAD

*1 cup fresh cauliflower, in bite-size pieces*
*½ cup pitted Kalamata olives*
*1 small purple onion, sliced*
*½ cup cooked garbanzo beans*
*2 small tomatoes, quartered*
*½ cup grated carrot or 2 carrots cut into thin strips*
*2 hard-boiled eggs, quartered*
*Goat or feta cheese chunks (or tofu)*
*3 cups leaf, romaine, or arugula lettuce, torn into small pieces*
*½ cup green or purple kale*

**Marinade:**
*½ cup olive oil*
*¼ cup vinegar*
*½ teaspoon sea salt*
*Pinch oregano*
*1 clove garlic, crushed*

Mix all marinade ingredients. Put cauliflower, olives, onion slices, and garbanzo beans in a dish and cover with the marinade. Refrigerate 8 hours or overnight. Drain and reserve marinade. Arrange vegetables over lettuce pieces and add remaining ingredients. Toss lightly. Cover with remaining marinade or your favorite vinaigrette dressing.

## POTATO SALAD

*6 or 7 medium potatoes*
*1 medium onion, chopped*
*2 hard-boiled eggs, sliced*
*½ cup safflower mayonnaise*
*1 teaspoon sea salt*
*¼ cup sunflower seeds*

Cook potatoes in their skins, then pare and dice into bite-size pieces. Add onion, eggs, mayonnaise, and salt. Mix gently. Sprinkle sunflower seeds over the top and chill well before serving. This is a very refreshing summer salad.

## SUMMER SALAD DRESSING

*1 tomato, quartered*
*1 cucumber, peeled and quartered*
*2 green onions, or 2 tablespoons chives, chopped*
*½ cup oil*
*2 tablespoons red wine vinegar*
*⅛ teaspoon sea salt*
*1 clove garlic, chopped*

Blend all ingredients in the blender and chill 1 hour. Pour over tossed salad and enjoy.

## APPLE SALAD

*Apple, chopped*

*Celery, chopped*
*Walnuts, chopped or in pieces*
*Raisins*
*Yogurt*

Gently combine apples, celery, walnuts, and raisins in a small bowl. Add yogurt and chill for 1 hour.

## KALE CHIPS

*2 cups kale, washed, dried, and stems removed*
*1 tablespoon extra virgin olive oil*
*Sprinkle of lime juice (optional)*
*Sea salt to taste*

Preheat oven to 250°F while preparing kale. Toss kale in a bowl with the olive oil and salt to coat the greens. Bake for about 30-40 minutes. Gently flip kale leaves several times during baking and watch closely so they don't burn.

## OVEN-ROASTED GREEN BEANS

*1 pound fresh green beans*
*2 tablespoons olive oil*
*1 clove garlic, crushed (optional)*
*½ teaspoon salt*

Preheat over to 425°F. Wash and trim the stems from the green beans. Place in a large bowl and toss with oil, salt, and garlic. Spread over a baking sheet and pop in the oven. Bake in the oven for 12-15 minutes.

## SPINACH DIP

*1 large bunch of spinach (about 1 pound), lightly steamed*
*½ cup green onions, chopped*

*1 tablespoon parsley (optional)*
*½ teaspoon dill weed*
*1 cup yogurt or sour cream*
*1 cup safflower mayonnaise*
*1 tablespoon lemon juice*
*¼ teaspoon chives*
*Dash thyme*
*¼ teaspoon sea salt*

Blend all ingredients in blender. Chill in refrigerator overnight. Serve with your favorite fresh vegetables.

## VEGGIE PLATTER

*Broccoli florets*
*Cauliflowerettes*
*Carrot sticks*
*Sugar snap peas*
*Celery sticks*
*Green onions*
*Cherry tomatoes*
*Zucchini pieces*
*Mushroom slices*
*Radishes (a variety of Daikon, spring, French breakfast, and Easter egg radishes provide color and pleasure to the plate.)*

Wash and prepare vegetables and arrange on a bed of lettuce. Serve with spinach dip or your favorite hummus dip.

## GUACAMOLE

*1 ripe avocado*
*1 tablespoon lemon juice*
*1 small tomato, diced*
*1 clove garlic, crushed*
*½ teaspoon chili powder*

*Dash Tabasco sauce*

Mash avocado with a fork. Add remaining ingredients and blend well. Chill 1 hour and serve with tortilla chips.

## LENTIL SOUP

*2 cloves garlic, chopped*
*1 large onion, chopped*
*1 large carrot, grated*
*2 large potatoes, chopped small*
*2 tablespoons oil*
*1 cup washed lentils*
*3 cups tomato juice or 1 large (28 ounce) can diced tomatoes*
*3 cups water or stock*
*Thyme*
*Sea salt*
*Optional: corn, peas, grated cheese*

Sauté garlic, onion, carrot, and potatoes in oil on low heat. Add remaining ingredients (adding thyme and salt, to taste). Bring to a boil, then simmer 1 hour. Top with grated cheese.

This is one of our favorite soup recipes. If you've never tried lentils before, this is the perfect recipe to quickly learn to like this little bean! Serve with salad, hearty bread, or corn tortillas. This makes a wonderful fall or winter meal.

## ROASTED CAULIFLOWER SOUP

*1 head cauliflower*
*2 medium potatoes, chopped*
*1 clove garlic, minced*
*1 shallot, finely chopped*
*1 carrot, grated*
*1 tablespoon olive oil*

3 cups vegetable broth
Sea salt and pepper

Preheat over to 350°F while chopping vegetables. Chop the cauliflower into 1-inch pieces and place in a bowl. Add potatoes, garlic, shallots, and carrot. Drizzle the olive oil over the top and stir to coat vegetables. Place on a baking pan and bake for 25 minutes.

Spoon 1 cup of the roasted vegetables at a time into a blender. Add 1 cup of broth and blend quickly (just a few seconds). If you blend until pureed, the potatoes will be sticky, so when in doubt, have the mixture more choppy than smooth. Repeat until all is blended. Add remaining broth, salt, and pepper and simmer for 20 minutes. Enjoy!

## POTATO SOUP

1 onion, chopped
3 carrots, grated
1 stalk celery, chopped
7-8 red potatoes, diced (wash well and leave skins on if organic)
¼ cup oil
1 quart stock or water
1 teaspoon salt
1½ cups non-instant dry milk
½ cup milk
Grated cheddar cheese (optional)
Chives, chopped (optional)

Sauté onion, carrots, celery, and potatoes in oil on low heat until tender. Pour in stock and add vegetable salt. Bring to boil, then simmer 1 hour or cook 15 minutes in a pressure cooker. Add dry milk powder to 2 cups of soup liquid and 1/2 cup milk and blend quickly in blender until milk powder is dissolved. Blending quickly is key; otherwise the soup turns to a sticky, thick, starchy texture. Add to the soup and simmer 5 minutes. Serve topped with grated cheddar cheese or a sprinkling of chopped chives. Serves 4.

## CUCUMBER SOUP

*4 cups cucumber, chopped*
*2 cups water*
*2 cups yogurt or sour cream or combination*
*1 clove garlic, minced*
*1 tablespoon honey*
*1 teaspoon sea salt*
*¼ teaspoon dill*
*1 green onion, chopped*

Put all ingredients into blender or food processor and puree. Chill and serve. Serves 4.

## MISO SOUP

*1 zucchini, sliced*
*1 carrot, grated*
*1 clove garlic, chopped*
*1 small onion, chopped*
*4 or 5 mushrooms, sliced*
*1 tablespoon olive oil*
*2 tablespoons miso (the garbanzo-flavored miso is a favorite)*
*4 cups water*
*1 teaspoon red wine vinegar*
*½ teaspoon honey*
*¼ teaspoon sesame oil*
*4 ounces tofu, cut in cubes*
*¼ cup scallions, chopped*

Sauté zucchini, carrot, garlic, onion, and mushrooms in oil. In a bowl, dissolve miso in water. Add to cooked vegetables. Gently stir in vinegar, honey, and sesame oil. Cover and simmer gently for 15 minutes. Add tofu and simmer one more minute. Sprinkle in the scallions and serve. Makes 2-3 servings.

# FAMILY PIZZA

### Crust:
*1 tablespoon dry yeast*
*1½ cups warm water*
*1 teaspoon honey*
*2 tablespoons oil*
*1½ teaspoons sea salt*
*3-3½ cups flour*

### Sauce:
*2 cloves garlic, chopped*
*1 large onion, chopped*
*1 carrot, finely grated*
*¼ cup grated zucchini (optional)*
*½ green pepper, chopped (optional)*
*2 tablespoons olive oil*
*1 28-ounce can tomatoes*
*1 12-ounce can tomato puree*
*Oregano, basil, salt, and pepper, to taste*
*½ teaspoon baking soda*

### Cheese:
*Mozzarella, shredded*
*Provolone, shredded*
*Sprinkle of Parmesan*

Dissolve yeast in water with honey. When yeast makes bubbles on surface, add oil and salt. Add flour a bit at a time, enough to make stiff dough. Knead 10 minutes and let rise 1½ hours.

Sauté garlic, onion, and other vegetables in oil. Add remaining sauce ingredients except baking soda. Bring to a boil, then sprinkle on baking soda and stir in. Simmer 1-2 hours.

Punch dough down and spread out on two oiled pizza pans. Spread with sauce and add cheeses. Bake 15 minutes in preheated 425°F oven.

## MOLLY'S TASTY TORTILLAS

(A great favorite with teenagers)

*4 whole wheat or corn tortillas*
*1½ cups cheese, grated*
*Arugula or Romaine lettuce*
*Tomato slices (optional)*

Divide ingredients evenly over each tortilla. Broil for 5-10 minutes, until cheese melts. Take them out of the oven, roll them up, and enjoy!

## ABU'S VEGETARIAN SUSHI

*1 package of nori (seaweed)*
*Thinly sliced cucumber (carrots, avocado, or any other fun veggies—experiment!)*
*1 cup sticky, white sushi rice*
*(Optional: Add 1 tablespoon Ume Plum Vinegar and 1 teaspoon honey to cooking rice)*
*Small bowl of water*
*Tamari for dipping*

Special note: This recipe was created by my 15-year-old grandson and is in his own words.

"Lay the nori onto a bamboo mat. Spread a thin layer of rice onto the nori, leaving one thin edge free of rice. Place the sliced veggies on top of the rice along the opposite edge. Pick up the mat at the veggies side and begin rolling tightly. Dipping your fingers into the water, dampen the other edge of the nori to help seal it together (this takes a little practice, but it's easy once you get a feel for it). Dip in the tamari and enjoy!"

## CALZONE

**Dough:**
*1 tablespoon yeast*

*2 tablespoons honey*
*2 cups warm water*
*1 tablespoon salt*
*5½-6 cups flour*

**Filling:**
*2 cloves garlic, crushed*
*½ cup minced onion*
*1 tablespoon olive oil*
*1 pound lightly steamed spinach*
*1 tablespoon water*
*1 pound ricotta cheese*
*2 cups grated mozzarella cheese*
*½ cup grated Parmesan cheese*
*Salt*
*Pepper*
*Dash of nutmeg*

**After baked:**
*A bit of butter*

**Dough**: Dissolve yeast in water with honey. Add salt and flour. Knead 10-15 minutes. Cover and set to rise 1 hour while you prepare filling.

**Filling:** Sauté garlic and onion in oil while steaming spinach in a steamer basket or in a skillet with a tablespoon of water. Drain spinach and place in a large bowl. Gently mix in the three cheeses with the spinach. Add the sautéed garlic and onion. Season with salt, pepper, and nutmeg, to taste.

**Now back to the dough:** When dough has risen, punch down and divide into 8-10 balls. Roll each ball out into a circle 1/4-inch thick. Fill with 1/2 to 3/4 cup filling. (Place filling on half of circle, fold over and make a 1/2-inch rim.) Moisten edges with water to help keep firmly closed. "Crimp" with a fork (by pressing down the tines all along the edges) and prick the top several times with the fork to let steam out during the baking. Bake on an oiled baking sheet at 450°F for 15-20 minutes. Brush with melted butter as soon as they come out of the oven. Makes 8-10 calzone. This is a very special meal and is great served with a tossed salad.

## SPAGHETTI SAUCE

*2 cloves garlic, chopped*
*1 large onion, chopped*
*1 stalk celery, chopped*
*1 large carrot, grated*
*½ zucchini, grated*
*2 tablespoons olive oil*
*1 28-ounce can tomatoes*
*1 16-ounce can tomato sauce*
*1 6-ounce can tomato paste*
*½ cup water*
*Oregano, basil, salt, and pepper, to taste*

Sauté the first five ingredients in oil until onions are translucent. Add remaining ingredients and season, to taste. Simmer 2-3 hours. Add mushrooms during the last half hour if you wish. Don't let the carrots and zucchini scare you away from this recipe. They add a lot of vitamins and fullness to the sauce, and it tastes almost the same as regular spaghetti sauce.

## SPAGHETTI SQUASH

*1 large spaghetti squash*
*1 quart spaghetti sauce*

Wash squash and pat dry with a towel. Pierce the skin of the squash several times with the point of a knife or the tines of a fork. Place on a cookie sheet and bake at 350°F for 1¼-1½ hours. Test for tenderness by piercing with a fork. Do not overcook. Remove squash from the oven and cut lengthwise. Gently scoop out "spaghetti" strands and place in a large bowl. Cover with your favorite spaghetti sauce or sautéed vegetables and sprinkle with grated Parmesan cheese. Add your favorite greens to create a delightful dinner everyone will enjoy! This is a great gluten-free dish.

# LASAGNA

*1 pound lasagna noodles*
*16 ounces ricotta cheese or tofu or a mixture of both*
*2 eggs*
*Dash cinnamon*
*Dash nutmeg*
*½ teaspoon parsley (optional)*
*2 cups shredded mozzarella cheese*
*1½-2 quarts spaghetti sauce*
*Grated Parmesan cheese*

Cook lasagna noodles while preparing cheeses. In a large bowl, combine ricotta cheese, eggs, cinnamon, nutmeg, and parsley and mix well. Set aside. Shred mozzarella cheese and place in another bowl. Have spaghetti sauce ready. Preheat oven to 350°F. In a large, flat baking dish (oblong cake pans work well), place a layer of sauce, a layer of noodles, and the ricotta cheese mixture (spread evenly over noodles). Continue with a layer of sauce, another layer of noodles, a layer of mozzarella cheese, a layer of sauce, and another layer of noodles. Finish with more sauce, then sprinkle the top with Parmesan cheese. Bake at 350°F for 45 minutes. Cool 15 minutes before cutting.

**Spinach Lasagna:** Follow above recipe but add a layer of steamed spinach (about a half pound) and 1/4 cup sautéed chopped onions or shallots. Sprinkle 1/4 cup Parmesan cheese over the spinach layer before adding the sauce.

## EGGPLANT PARMESAN

*1 medium eggplant*
*⅓ cup whole wheat flour*
*½ teaspoon sea salt*
*⅛ teaspoon cayenne pepper*
*1 tablespoon grated Parmesan cheese*
*2 tablespoons whole wheat bread crumbs*
*¼ teaspoon dried parsley or 1 teaspoon fresh parsley, chopped*
*1 egg*
*2 tablespoons milk*
*2 tablespoons olive oil*
*2 cups spaghetti sauce*
*1 cup shredded mozzarella cheese*
*¼ cup finely grated Parmesan cheese*

Slice eggplant into 1/2-inch slices. Combine flour, salt, cayenne pepper, 1 tablespoon Parmesan cheese, bread crumbs, and parsley. Mix egg and milk in a small bowl. Dip each eggplant slice into egg mixture, flour the eggplant, and then place slices in oiled skillet. Sauté eggplant until lightly browned on each side, then drain slices on a paper towel. Arrange eggplant on a baking dish over one-half the spaghetti sauce. Pour remaining sauce over the top; then sprinkle with mozzarella and Parmesan cheeses. Bake at 350°F for 20-30 minutes. Serves 4.

## SPINACH SEASHELLS

*¼ cup chopped onion*
*1 clove garlic, crushed*
*1 tablespoon oil*
*1 pound fresh, washed spinach, chopped*
*1 pound ricotta cheese*
*10 ounces mozzarella cheese, shredded*
*⅓ cup grated Parmesan cheese*
*2 eggs, beaten*
*1 teaspoon sea salt*
*½ teaspoon oregano*

*8 ounces large seashell pasta*
*1 quart spaghetti sauce*

Sauté onion and garlic in oil until soft. Add spinach and steam lightly. In large bowl, combine cheeses, eggs, salt, and oregano. Gently stir in drained spinach mixture. Fill shells with spinach-cheese mixture and arrange in oiled baking dish (9" x 13"). Cover with spaghetti sauce. Bake at 350°F for 40 minutes. Serves 4.

## ENCHILADA BAKE

*1 small onion, chopped*
*1 clove garlic, crushed*
*½ green pepper, chopped*
*½ cup mushrooms, sliced (optional)*
*3 tablespoons oil*
*1 28-ounce can whole tomatoes*
*1 teaspoon ground cumin (optional)*
*2 teaspoons chili powder*
*½ teaspoon salt*
*6 corn tortillas*
*1½-2 cups cooked black (turtle) beans*
*1 cup ricotta cheese or ½ cup ricotta and ½ cup tofu*
*1 cup shredded Monterey Jack cheese*
*Black olives, sliced (optional)*

Sauté onion, garlic, green pepper, and mushrooms in the oil. Add tomatoes, cumin, chili powder, and salt to make the sauce. Simmer for 30 minutes. Line an oiled casserole dish with three corn tortillas, half of the beans, half of the sauce, half of the ricotta, and half of the Monterey Jack cheese. Repeat layers. Sprinkle sliced olives over the top. Bake uncovered at 350°F for 20 minutes.

## MEXICAN POTATO BAKE

*4 baked potatoes*

*2 cups refried black beans*
*1 cup shredded Cheddar cheese*

Cut baked potatoes lengthwise. Place 1/2 cup of the beans on each potato, then top with 1/4 cup cheese. Return to the oven for 5 minutes until the cheese melts.

## BROCCOLI QUICHE

*Pastry for 9-inch pie*
*1 cup grated Swiss cheese*
*1 tablespoon onion, finely chopped*
*1 cup steamed broccoli, cut into bite-size pieces*
*¼ cup roasted red peppers, chopped*
*¼ cup sautéed mushrooms (optional)*
*4 eggs*
*1¾ cups cream or milk*
*½ teaspoon sea salt*
*½ teaspoon cayenne pepper*
*¼ teaspoon honey*

Prepare pastry and line a 9-inch pie pan or quiche dish. Sprinkle cheese, onion, broccoli, red peppers, and mushrooms into pie pan. Beat eggs with a fork, add remaining ingredients to eggs and mix gently. Pour into pie pan. Bake 15 minutes at 425°F, then 30 minutes at 300°F. Quiche is done when a knife inserted 1 inch from the edge comes out clean. Let quiche stand 10 minutes before cutting. This is excellent served with a salad.

## CRUSTLESS QUICHE

*½ cup sliced mushrooms*
*½ cup chopped onion*
*1 zucchini, chopped*
*1 clove garlic, chopped*
*2 tablespoons oil*

*5 eggs*
*½ cup milk*
*½ teaspoon sea salt*
*4 ounces goat cheese, crumbled*
*1 cup grated Cheddar cheese*
*1 cup whole wheat bread cubes*

Sauté mushrooms, onion, zucchini, and garlic in oil for 5 minutes. Combine eggs, milk, and salt in a small bowl and mix lightly. Gently stir in cheese then add bread cubes. Pour into oiled 9-inch pie pan. Bake at 350°F for 45 minutes. Let stand 5 minutes before serving. Serves 4.

## FALAFEL BURGERS

*¼ cup onion, chopped*
*1 clove garlic, crushed*
*2 tablespoons olive oil*
*2 cups cooked garbanzo beans*
*2 potatoes, cooked*
*2 tablespoons sesame butter*
*1 tablespoon lemon juice*
*1 tablespoon non-instant dry milk*
*2 teaspoons soy sauce*
*1 tablespoon chopped parsley (optional)*
*½ teaspoon chili powder (optional)*

**Top with:**
*Lettuce pieces*
*Tomato, sliced*
*Cucumber, sliced*

Sauté onion and garlic in oil. Mash garbanzo beans and potatoes with a fork or puree in blender or food processor. Add sautéed onion and garlic, sesame butter, lemon juice, dry milk, soy sauce, parsley, and chili powder.

Shape into patties and place on oiled cookie sheet. Bake in 350°F oven, 10 minutes on each side. Serve in pita bread with lettuce, tomato, and cucumber. Sesame seed dressing can be drizzled over sandwich for added flavor. This recipe can also be made into garbanzo balls for and served as an appetizers.

## CABBAGE, ZUCCHINI, & TOMATO BAKE

*½ cup onion, chopped*
*1 tablespoon olive oil*
*1 head cabbage, chopped*
*2 zucchini, chopped*
*1 28-ounce can tomatoes*

Sauté onion in oil until soft. Add cabbage and zucchini and steam for 10 minutes. (Add a bit of water to help steaming process if necessary.) Add tomatoes. Turn into lightly oiled casserole dish and bake 45 minutes in 350°F oven.

## ZUCCHINI CHEESE BAKE

*2 medium zucchini, sliced*
*2 large tomatoes, chopped*
*1 16-ounce can tomato sauce*
*½ teaspoon thyme*
*½ cup shredded provolone*
*1 clove garlic, minced*

Combine all ingredients in an oiled baking dish. Bake at 350°F for 45 minutes. Serves 4.

## STUFFED BAKED ZUCCHINI WITH QUINOA

*2 medium zucchini*
*½ cup chopped onion*
*2 tablespoons olive oil*

½ *cup sunflower seeds, chopped*
¾ *cup yogurt*
2 *teaspoons lemon juice*
¼ *teaspoon sea salt*
½ *cup cooked brown rice, quinoa, or bulgur*
½ *teaspoon chopped parsley*
1 *tomato, chopped*

Slice zucchini in half and scoop out the center, leaving a firm shell. Reserve the inside pulp. Sauté onion in oil until soft. Add the zucchini pulp and cook for 5 minutes. Add remaining ingredients and cook 5 more minutes. Spoon mixture back into zucchini shells and bake at 350°F for 20-30 minutes.

## SARAH'S BAKED ZUCCHINI WITH GOAT CHEESE

4 *large zucchini*
1 *tablespoon olive oil*
2 *tablespoons chopped onion*
¼ *cup crushed almonds*
*Salt and pepper, to taste*
¾ *cup cooked bulgur or quinoa*
1 *cup goat cheese pieces (or feta)*

Preheat oven to 425°F. Hollow out the inside of the zucchini (you can do this with a spoon). Chop zucchini into bite size pieces. Set aside. Sauté onion in olive oil over low heat. Add zucchini and cook over medium heat for 5 minutes. Gently stir in almonds, bulgur or quinoa, and cheese. Scoop mixture into the hollowed-out zucchini and bake for about 20-25 minutes. Serve with lemon slices.

## CREAMY SPINACH

2 *tablespoons butter*
2 *tablespoons flour*
1½ *cups milk*

*Dash cayenne pepper*
*⅛ teaspoon nutmeg*
*½ cup Parmesan cheese or tofu (finely chopped)*
*1 pound fresh spinach, chopped*
*1 small onion, chopped*
*1 tablespoon olive oil*

Make a white sauce with the first six ingredients by melting butter in a saucepan, then adding flour to make a paste. Slowly add milk and mix with a wire whip or a wooden spoon. Add cayenne and nutmeg. Simmer 2 minutes. Pour over steamed spinach.

**To steam spinach:** Wash spinach and drain well. Sauté onion in oil for 3 minutes, then add spinach and steam for 3 more minutes.

## ZACHARY'S PEANUT BUTTER BALLS

(From Zack's early kitchen adventures and in his own words . . .)

*1 cup peanut butter*
*½ cup dry milk (not instant kind)*
*Some wheat germ (Mom says about ½ cup)*
*Some sesame seeds (about ⅓ cup)*
*¼ cup honey*
*Dash of vanilla*

"Mix everything up all together real good. Roll them up into little balls. Put them in the refrigerator. Yummy! You can put raisins in them; my sister likes them like that, but I don't."

**Variations:**
Add 1/4 cup carob chips or cacao nibs. Instead of shaping into balls, press mixture into a square baking dish. Chill. Cut into bars.

# CAITLIN'S BERRIES & CREAM

*1 cup berries (strawberries, blackberries, blueberries, or raspberries)*
*½ cup cream or creamy Greek yogurt*
*1 tablespoon honey*
*½ teaspoon vanilla extract*

Wash berries and place them in a small bowl. Mix cream, honey, and vanilla together and pour over berries. Enjoy!

# RED, WHITE, AND BLUE SPECIAL

*Frozen yogurt*
*Blueberries*
*Strawberries*
*Whipped cream*

Cover yogurt with fruit and top with whipped cream.

# TROPICAL BANANA SUNDAE

*1 banana, sliced*
*1 tablespoon shredded fresh coconut*
*¼ cup milk or yogurt*
*1 tablespoon honey*
*Dash cinnamon*
*Blueberries*

Mix all ingredients together in a small bowl. Top with blueberries. Serves 1.

# WARM CACAO WITH CINNAMON

*2 cups almond milk*
*3 tablespoons cacao nibs or cacao powder*
*A bit of liquid stevia to taste*

Combine all ingredients in a blender. Heat and stir in a pan on the stovetop. Enjoy!

## ORANGE-STRAWBERRY PUNCH

*1 quart orange juice*
*½ apple, cored and pared*
*1 tablespoon lemon juice*
*¼ cup strawberries*
*1 tablespoon honey*

Blend all ingredients in a blender and serve over ice. Serves 4.

## ZACHARY'S OWN SHAKE

*1½ cups milk*
*1 tablespoon carob powder*
*1 tablespoon honey*
*I banana*
*¼ teaspoon lecithin*
*¼ teaspoon vanilla extract*
*2 tablespoons peanut butter*

Mix all ingredients in blender on high speed until smooth and creamy. (This recipe was truly invented by Zack when he was eight years old.)

## TAMARI NUT MIX

*2 cups sunflower seeds*
*1 cup pumpkin seeds*
*½ cup tamari sauce*

Mix seeds with tamari sauce and let stand for 30 minutes. Bake on a baking sheet at 300°F for 15 minutes and stir twice. Cool and store in airtight container. Delicious served with your favorite sandwich or for an afternoon snack.

# FRUIT LEATHER

*1 pound very ripe fruit (apples, apricots, peaches, pears, or strawberries)*
*1 tablespoon honey*

Wash, peel, and core fruit. Place fruit in blender or food processor and blend. Pour into saucepan, add honey, and heat mixture just until it boils, stirring frequently. Cook for 3 minutes. Line cookie sheets with a layer of plastic wrap. Pour fruit onto plastic and spread into a thin layer. Carefully stretch a layer of cheesecloth over tray, being careful to keep it off the fruit mixture. Place tray in the sun for about 8 hours (or place in electric oven on lowest heat). Fruit leather is done when it can be peeled away from plastic wrap. This is a wonderful, natural, preservative-free treat everyone will love!

# SUPER YUMMY NUT & BERRY MIX

*Walnuts*
*Shredded coconut*
*Raisins*
*Gogi berries or dried cranberries*

Toss together and enjoy.

# BANANA PUDDING

*¼ cup unsweetened almond milk*
*2 tablespoons unsweetened cocoa powder*
*3 ripe bananas*
*1 teaspoon vanilla extract*
*A bit of honey or stevia, to taste*

Blend quickly in blender. Chill. Served topped with a sprinkling of cacao nibs.

## VEGAN NO-BAKE PROTEIN BARS
(That even non-vegans love!)

*1½ cups whole oats*
*½ cup shredded coconut*
*½ cup pumpkin seeds*
*¼ cup raw sesame seeds*
*½ cup dried fruit (raisins, cranberries, cherries, apricots, gogi berries, date pieces, etc.)*
*¼ cup maple syrup*
*1 teaspoon vanilla*
*½ cup peanut butter (or any nut butter)*
*¼ cup brown rice powder or garbanzo bean flour*
*2 tablespoons ground flax seeds*
*1 tablespoon chia seeds (optional)*
*1½ teaspoons cinnamon*
*1 teaspoon vanilla extract*
*⅓ cup warm water (judge the texture you want)*

Toss in a handful of cacao nibs if you like.

Mix all dry ingredients together. Press into an 8" x 8" inch dish. (The mixture will be sticky but fun to taste before it goes into the fridge!) Cover and refrigerate until firm. Cut into individual servings and enjoy. Keeps for about 2 weeks in the refrigerator, or wrap individually and freeze.

*Chapter Thirteen*

# RECIPES FOR A CHILD
# WITH ALLERGIES

The following recipes offer ideas for the parents coping with nutritional needs of a child with allergies. These recipes are free of one or all of the following common food allergens: eggs, milk, wheat, and gluten. Be sure to check ingredients in recipes in all other sections of this book and substitute and adapt where necessary. Although this is mentioned in chapter 7, it feels right to repeat it here. Look closely at the labels if your child has these sensitivities or allergies.

## SQUASH MILK

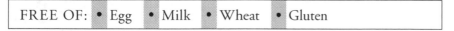

| FREE OF: | • Egg | • Milk | • Wheat | • Gluten |
| --- | --- | --- | --- | --- |

*1 yellow squash, diced*
*¼ cup water*

Dice and remove the seeds from a medium-size yellow summer squash (but don't peel it). Measure 1¼ cups of the squash into blender jar. Pour in water just to cover the squash. Whirl in blender on high speed until smooth, 1-2 minutes. Strain. Makes about 1 cup. Good for baking, especially in spice cake or pumpkin pie.

## BANANA SHAKE

| FREE OF: | • Egg | • Milk | • Wheat | • Gluten |
|----------|-------|--------|---------|----------|

*1½ cups nut milk*
*1 banana*
*Dash vanilla extract*

Blend in blender at high speed until smooth.

## TOFU MAYONNAISE

| FREE OF: | • Egg | Milk | • Wheat | • Gluten |
|----------|-------|------|---------|----------|

*8 ounces tofu*
*2 tablespoons cider vinegar*
*½ cup yogurt*
*1 tablespoon fresh lemon juice*
*1 teaspoon gluten-free tamari*
*1 tablespoon oil (sunflower or olive)*
*½ teaspoon dry mustard*
*1 clove garlic, minced (optional)*

Puree all ingredients in blender or food processor until smooth. Store in jar with tight-fitting lid. Keeps in refrigerator for 1 week. Makes 1½ cups mayonnaise.

## TOFU DIP

| FREE OF: | • Egg | • Milk | • Wheat | • Gluten |
|----------|-------|--------|---------|----------|

*8 ounces tofu, drained*
*4 teaspoons fresh lemon juice*
*1 teaspoon onion juice or 1 clove garlic, minced*
*¼ teaspoon dry mustard*
*¼ teaspoon sea salt*

*⅛ teaspoon celery seeds*

Drain tofu well. Blend all ingredients in blender. Chill 1 hour. Good as a dip for vegetables and crackers and as a sour cream substitute.

## PEANUT BUTTER-TOFU DELUXE

| FREE OF: | • Egg | • Milk | • Wheat | • Gluten |
|----------|-------|--------|---------|----------|

*8 ounces tofu, drained*
*½ cup peanut butter*
*1 tablespoon honey*
*1 banana, mashed*
*¼ cup sunflower seeds, chopped (optional)*
*¼ cup raisins (optional)*

Blend tofu, peanut butter, honey, and banana in blender or food processor. Add sunflower seeds and raisins if desired. Great on rice cakes or gluten-free crackers.

## JOSH'S TOFU PANCAKES

| FREE OF: | • Egg | • Milk | Wheat | Gluten |
|----------|-------|--------|-------|--------|

*¼ cup crumbled tofu*
*1½ cups water*
*1 tablespoon maple syrup*
*1 teaspoon vanilla extract*
*¼ cup oil*
*1½ cups whole wheat flour*
*1½ teaspoons baking powder*

Blend tofu and liquid ingredients in blender until smooth. Mix flour and baking powder in medium bowl. Stir in liquid ingredients, mixing gently just until the dry ingredients are moistened. Grease and heat a griddle or skillet. Drop batter from a large spoon onto griddle, lightly spreading each cake with the back of a spoon to make a round cake. Cook until bottom of pancake is golden brown and edges of pancake begin to look dry. With spatula or pancake turner, loosen and turn cake, and brown other side. Serve at once with maple syrup or apple butter.

## BUCKWHEAT PANCAKES

| FREE OF: | Egg | • Milk | • Wheat | • Gluten |
|----------|-----|--------|---------|----------|

*1½ cups buckwheat flour*
*2½ teaspoons corn-free, gluten-free baking powder*
*½ teaspoon sea salt*
*¼ cup sunflower oil*
*¾ cup water*
*2 eggs, beaten*
*2 tablespoons honey*

Combine all dry ingredients in a large bowl. Mix together oil, water, eggs, and honey. Stir liquid ingredients into the dry ingredients. Pour batter onto oiled griddle or skillet. Flip when brown on one side. Serves 3-4.

## RICE PANCAKES

| FREE OF: | • Egg | • Milk | • Wheat | • Gluten |
|----------|-------|--------|---------|----------|

*2 cups cooked brown rice*
*2 cups tofu, drained and chopped*
*2 tablespoons lemon juice*
*1 teaspoon sea salt*
*2 tablespoons potato flour*
*¼ cup chopped walnuts (optional)*

Mix rice and tofu together in a large bowl. Add remaining ingredients. Shape into 4-6 pancakes and cook in oiled skillet. Cook until golden on both sides.

# RICE WAFFLES

| FREE OF: | Egg | • Milk | • Wheat | • Gluten |
|---|---|---|---|---|

*2 cups rice flour*
*2 cups rice milk (free of casein, sodium caseinate, or lactalbumin)*
*4 teaspoons corn-free, gluten-free baking powder*
*½ teaspoon sea salt*
*¼ cup oil*
*2 eggs, separated*

Mix all dry ingredients in a large bowl. Gently mix egg yolks with a fork, then add the milk and oil to the egg yolks. Stir into dry ingredients. Beat egg whites until stiff and gently fold into batter. Cook on lightly oiled skillet or griddle. Serves 4.

# RYE BREAD

| FREE OF: | • Egg | • Milk | • Wheat | Gluten |
|---|---|---|---|---|

*1 tablespoon dry yeast*
*1¼ cups warm water*
*1 teaspoon honey*
*2 tablespoons safflower or olive oil*
*4 cups rye flour*
*2 teaspoons salt*
*3 tablespoons caraway seeds (optional)*

Dissolve yeast with water and honey. Add oil. Stir in dry ingredients, adding more water if necessary. Knead 10 minutes. Cover and let rise in a warm place for 1½ hours. Punch down. Knead 5 minutes, shape into 1 loaf, and place in oiled bread pan. Cover and let rise 30 minutes. Bake 1 hour and 10 minutes at 375°F.

## WONDERFUL WHEAT BERRY BREAD

| FREE OF: | • Egg | • Milk | Wheat | Gluten |
|---|---|---|---|---|

*¾ cup whole wheat berries*
*2 cups water*
*1 cup whole wheat flour*
*1 cup chopped nuts*
*1 teaspoon baking soda*
*1 teaspoon sea salt*
*½ cup crumbled tofu*
*½ cup water*
*¼ cup barley malt or maple syrup*
*2 tablespoons oil*

Combine whole wheat berries and water in medium saucepan. Bring to boil over medium heat and boil for 2 minutes. Turn off heat, cover saucepan, and let stand for 1-2 hours. Bring to boil again and simmer, uncovered for 1½ hours or until tender.

Preheat oven to 350°F. Mix flour, nuts, baking soda and salt in a large bowl. Place tofu, water, barley malt or maple syrup, and oil in blender and blend until smooth. Stir tofu mixture into flour mixture and mix just until dry ingredients are moistened. Drain wheat berries and fold into bread mixture. Pour into oiled bread pan. Bake 1 hour. Let cool in pan for 10 minutes, then turn out on wire rack to finish cooling.

## BANANA NUT BREAD

| FREE OF: | Egg | • Milk | • Wheat | • Gluten |
|---|---|---|---|---|

*1½ cups banana, mashed*
*2 tablespoons water*
*2 eggs*
*1½ cups arrowroot flour*
*1 teaspoon baking soda*

*½ teaspoon sea salt*
*¾ cup chopped walnuts*

Combine banana and water in a large bowl. Beat eggs, and then mix with banana. Stir in dry ingredients and mix well. Add chopped nuts. Bake at 350°F for 45 minutes in a lightly oiled bread pan.

## PEANUT BUTTER CAROB FUDGE

| FREE OF: | • Egg | Milk | • Wheat | Gluten |
|---|---|---|---|---|

*1 cup peanut butter*
*¾ cup honey*
*¾ cup toasted carob powder*
*¾ cup non-instant dry milk powder*

Mix all ingredients together with a fork, and then knead about 3 minutes to thoroughly combine mixture. Press into a 9" x 9" square pan and refrigerate several hours or overnight. Cut into squares and serve. Raisins can be added for a variation.

## BANANA-OAT CAKE

| FREE OF: | Egg | • Milk | • Wheat | • Gluten |
|---|---|---|---|---|

*2 cups oat flour (or ground, gluten-free oats)*
*2 teaspoons corn-free, gluten-free baking powder*
*½ teaspoon sea salt*
*2 tablespoons safflower oil*
*2 eggs*
*⅓ cup honey*
*2 tablespoons water*
*2-3 bananas, mashed*

Sift oat flour before measuring, and then sift with baking powder and salt. Beat oil, eggs, honey, and water in a small bowl. Add mashed banana to egg mixture and mix well. Combine liquid and dry ingredients. Pour into oiled 8" x 8" square pan and bake at 350°F for 30 minutes.

## OATMEAL SHEET CAKE

FREE OF: • Egg • Milk • Wheat • Gluten

*1 cup oat flour (or ground gluten-free oats)*
*1 tablespoon arrowroot*
*1 teaspoon cinnamon*
*1 teaspoon salt*
*½ teaspoon nutmeg*
*⅔ cup water*
*2 teaspoons corn-free, gluten-free baking powder*
*2 tablespoons safflower oil*
*1 banana, mashed*
*⅓ cup almonds or walnuts, chopped*
*¼ cup raisins*

Mix all ingredients in a large bowl. Pour into oiled 9" x 9" square baking pan. Bake at 350°F for 15-20 minutes.

*Chapter Fourteen*

# WHAT NOT TO PUT
# INTO THE MOUTHS
# OF BABES

Over five million children are poisoned each year in the United States. Globally, over 45,000 children and teens die from poisoning each year. Infants, toddlers, and children need not be out of sight long before they can inhale or ingest a toxic substance. Consider these facts about poisoning:

- Poisonings are most likely to occur in children under six years of age, with one-year-olds accounting for the highest number of poisonings reported. The American Association of Poison Control Centers reports calls about children under the age of six make up about 52% of all cases.
- There is an extremely high incidence of repeat poisonings. A child who is poisoned once probably will be poisoned again.
- A large number of ingested poisons are medications found within a child's reach or climb. (Give a toddler a chair, desk, toilet, or table to stand or climb on and he probably will.)
- Many first-aid antidote charts and labels are incorrect or out of date. Often a well-meaning parent does more harm than good by following directions from an old chart rather than phoning the Poison Control Center or a physician first. In fact, the old remedy of giving salt water to induce vomiting has even caused death.

- You may have poison-proofed your home but the homes of friends and relatives may have poisons within reach. Be especially cautious of this fact.

## IN AN EMERGENCY

Remain calm. The majority of poison emergencies can be resolved quickly.

### In the United States

**Call the Poison Center Hotline (1-800-222-1222):**

If you or another person has been poisoned, or think you may have been poisoned.

American Association of Poison Control Centers website: www.aapcc.org.

### Call 911:

If the person has collapsed, is unconscious, or has difficulty breathing.

### In Canada

**Call your local poison control center.**

Canadian Association of Poison Control Centers website: www.capcc.ca.

### Call 911:

If you have a poison emergency and your child has collapsed or is not breathing.

### Worldwide

World Health Organization directory of poison centers website: www. who.int.

**Important Update on Ipecac Syrup**
Beginning in the 1960s, parents were told to keep ipecac syrup available in case it's use was instructed by the Poison Control Center. This practice is no longer suggested since recent research has shown ipecac is not helpful and in fact, there are times when ipecac is unsafe. The American Academy of Pediatrics and the American Association of Poison Control Centers no longer recommend that parents keep ipecac syrup at home.

# FIRST AID FOR POISONING

## Swallowed Poisons

Call the poison center or your doctor. Call 911 if the person is unconscious, having difficulty breathing, agitated, or having seizures. Caution: Antidote charts and labels may be outdated and incorrect. Do not give salt, vinegar, mustard, raw eggs, or citrus juices.

## Inhaled Poisons

Immediately drag or carry the person to fresh air. Ventilate the area. Call the poison center.

## Poisons on the Skin

Remove contaminated clothing and rinse skin with water for five to ten minutes.
Wash gently with water and rinse.
Call the poison center.

## Poisons in the Eye

Flush the eye with lukewarm (not hot) low-pressure water for fifteen to twenty minutes. Water can be poured from a pitcher held two to three inches from the eye. You need not force the eyelid open, but have the person blink while flushing. Have someone call the Poison Control Center as soon as possible.

**Have this information ready when you call the Poison Control Center:**
Your name and phone number
Age and approximate weight of child
Name of product and ingredients
Amount ingested
The container
Symptoms
Time poisoning occurred
Any first aid already given

## POISON-PROOFING YOUR HOME

1.  Do you have the phone number of your local Poison Control Center and your physician in your cell phone and by your home phone(s)? If not, please put this book down and take two minutes to do that now. Circle these numbers for your babysitter. Your child is so precious!

> Don't ever hesitate to call the Poison Control Center if you think your child may have ingested or inhaled a possible poison. Early treatment can save a life.

2.  Store all medicines and household cleaning supplies out of reach (and sight) of infants and children. Use locked cabinets or child-resistant safety latches when necessary. Try to buy the least toxic cleaners and keep all products in their original containers.

3. Request child-resistant caps on all medicines (but don't assume that a child can't find a way to open them). Request extra child-resistant containers and transfer vitamins into them.

4. Never store medicine or any poisonous product in beverage or food containers. More than one unsuspecting child has picked up a soda bottle in the garage that was filled with gasoline or kerosene.

5. Never tell children that medicine tastes like candy or that foods you don't want them to eat or drink are "poison." Those unclear messages can cause confusion. For example, if too much medicine is taken because it tastes like candy, possible poisoning could be the result. It also is wise to take your own medicine when children aren't watching since they love to imitate grownups.

6. Check the dates of all drugs in your medicine cabinet and dispose of all old medicine. FDA guidelines for disposing unused medicine are simple. Take them out of their original container and mix them with used coffee grounds or kitty litter. Place them in a sealable bag or other container to prevent the medication from leaking or breaking out of a garbage bag. Dispose in household trash.

7. Keep vitamins and other supplements (even children's vitamins) out of reach. Iron, fluoride, or other poisoning could occur if a child ingests too many tablets or capsules. Do not let your child play with empty medicine bottles.

8. Remember to keep all potential poisons out of reach when your child is away from home.

9. Be aware of which plants in your home are poisonous.

According to the World Health Organization, the most common agents involved in childhood poisoning are:

- Over-the-counter medications
- Prescription medications and illicit drugs
- Vitamins and iron tablets
- Household products containing bleach, detergents, disinfectants, cleaning agents, vinegar
- Cosmetics
- Paraffin
- Kerosene
- Pesticides
- Poisonous plants

## Beware! The following products can cause poisoning:

aftershave lotion
alcohol
ammonia
antifreeze
aspirin
automatic dishwashing soaps
automotive products
bleach
charcoal lighter
ointments or creams
furniture polish
gasoline
glues and adhesives
hair dyes and bleaches
insecticides
jewelry containing beans or seeds
kerosene
lye

mothballs
mouthwash
nail polishes and removers
oven cleaners
paint and paint thinners
perfumes
pesticides
petroleum products
plants
plastics
rat poison
rubbing alcohol
shampoo and soap
toilet bowl cleaner
vitamins and minerals
weed killer

Other products also can be harmful. When in doubt, consult the Poison Control Center in your area. Keep your child safe. Put all poisons out of the reach of children.

~

# Closing Thoughts

So where do you want to go from here? You have the guidelines, recipes, and sacred nutrients at your fingertips. In the busyness of life that now includes a new little one (or more), you get to make the choices that you think are best. Please take the information in this book, keep what works for you, and leave the rest. Don't feel you need to offer your baby "perfect" food all the time. Do your best. Leave guilt out of the picture. If your mealtimes are filled with love, laughter, respect, and the best food choices you can make in that moment, pat yourself on the back. Let loving-kindness be the spice of your own precious intuition. And you can always expand the list of sacred nutrients to add to the food you serve. The list goes well beyond what is presented in this book.

You are invited to use *Into the Mouths of Babes* as a guide, a blueprint for creating nourishment for your child in the most joyful ways imaginable. To do that, you will need to be vigilant in taking good care of yourself. Mothers, especially, have been presented with centuries of modeling that often puts self-care in a category of selfish choices. I believe it is actually a "self-full" act, and that everyone around you is better for it when you practice self-care.

To close, I would like to offer you this gentle gift in the form of "The Voice of Self-Care." It is designed to be a loving support for mothers, fathers, grandparents, and all people caring for children. I wrote this "Voice of Self-Care" after being inspired by the writings of Debbie Rosas, co-creator of The Nia Technique.

I invite you to listen closely to that tenderly loving voice inside you. Change any words that don't resonate with you so you hear them as a loving voice you can embrace.

# The Voice of Self-Care

I am the voice of self-care, a knowing and wisdom available to all.

My job is to help you maintain wholeness, strength, and peace within so you can joyfully thrive.

I reorganize your relationship to living in a body so that you connect more deeply to love, joy, and your inner wisdom.

I am the voice that beckons you to care for yourself first, so you can then fully care for others—when that is your sacred task to perform.

I support you in consistently choosing acts of self-care.

I am the voice inside of you that beckons you to care for yourself with the love and intensity you would bestow upon a beloved child entrusted to your care.

I am the force that vibrates your trillions of cells into aligning to be you, as a whole human being, the whole you that you came to this Earth to be.

You sense me as the breath of your body breathing fully through you, as the beat of your heart pulsing in perfect rhythm—your senses delicious with anticipation of all that is nourishing.

Slow down and go inward and you can perceive my presence as a gentle friend standing next to you, offering constant and loving support—support that comes wholly and freely without a trace of judgment or criticism.

You have the ability to choose, seek, increase, and sustain the sacred acts of self-care, no matter what is going on in, or around, your life and world.

Choose me and you will sense a wholeness of body, mind, and spirit that over time will compel you, without thinking, to choose me again and again, until the path of self-care is the way you live.

~

Best wishes for happy feeding, growing, and loving times together.

-Susan

# Bibliography

Ballentine, Rudolph, M.D. *Diet and Nutrition: A Holistic Approach.* Honesdale, PA: Himalayan International Institute, 1979.

Brody, Jane E. *Jane Brody's Nutrition Book.* New York: Bantam Books, 1982.

Burkes, A. Wesley, M.D. et al. "Oral Immunotherapy for Treatment of Egg Allergy in Children." *New England Journal of Medicine* 367(2012); 233-243.

Castle, Sue. *The Complete New Guide to Preparing Baby Foods.* New York: Bantam, 1992.

Chopra, Deepak. *Quantum Healing: Exploring the Frontiers of Mind/Body Medicine.* New York: Bantam Books, 1989.

Colquhoun, James, and Laurentine ten Bosch. *Hungry for Change: Ditch the Diets, Conquer the Cravings, and Eat Your Way to Lifelong Health.* New York: HarperOne, 2012.

David, Marc. *The Slow Down Diet: Eating for Pleasure, Energy, & Weight Loss.* Rochester, VT: Healing Arts Press, 2005.

—. *Nourishing Wisdom: A Mind-Body Approach to Nutrition and Well-Being.* New York: Bell Tower, 1992.

Davis, Adelle. *Let's Cook It Right.* New York: NAL Dutton, 1988.

—. *Let's Get Well.* New York: NAL Dutton, 1972.

—. *Let's Have Healthy Children.* New York: NAL Dutton, 1981.

Dufty, William. *Sugar Blues.* New York: Warner Books, 1993.

Emerling, Carol G. and Eugene O. Jonckers. *The Allergy Cookbook: Delicious Recipes for Everyday and Special Occasions.* Garden City, NY: Doubleday & Company, 1969.

Ewald, Ellen. *Recipes for a Small Planet.* New York: Ballantine, 1985.

Feingold, Ben F. *Why Your Child Is Hyperactive.* New York: Random House, 1985.

Fields, Denise, and Ari Brown, M.D. *Baby 411.* Boulder, CO: Windsor Peak Press, 2013.

Flynn, Kathryn Simmons. *Cooking for Fertility.* Rosco, IL: The Fertile Soul, LLC, 2010.

Ford, Marjorie W., Susan Hillyard, and Mary Faulk Kooch. *The Deaf Smith Country Cookbook.* New York: Avery Publishers, 1991.

Friedman, Peach. *Diary of an Exercise Addict.* Guilford, CT: GPP Life, 2010.

Gaskin, Ina May. *Ina May's Guide to Childbirth.* New York: Bantam, 2003.

Goldbeck, Nikki, and David Goldbeck. *The Supermarket Handbook: Access to Whole Foods.* New York: NAL Dutton, 1976.

Golos, Natalie, and Frances Golos Golbitz. *Coping with Your Allergies.* New York: Simon and Schuster, 1986.

Gordon, Richard A. *Anorexia and Bulimia: Anatomy of a Social Epidemic.* Cambridge: Basil Blackwell, 1990.

Gorman, Christine. "Parents: Can the Juice!" *Time,* 11 April 1994, p. 64.

Hay, Louise L. *You Can Heal Your Life.* Farmingdale, New York: Coleman Publishing, 1984.

Harris, Mark. "Raising Healthy Veg Kids." *Vegetarian Times,* July 1994, pp. 58-65.

Hausman, Patricia, and Judith Benn Hurley. *The Healing Foods.* Emmaus, PA: Rodale Press, 1989.

Hirschfeld, Herman, M.D. *Understanding Your Allergy.* New York: Arco Publishing, 1979.

Holick, Michael F. *The Vitamin D Solution: A 3-Step Strategy to Cure Our Most Common Health Problems.* New York: Hudson Street Press, 2010.

—. "Vitamin D Deficiency." *New England Journal of Medicine* 357(2007): 266-81.

Houben, Milton, and William Kropf, M.D. *Harmful Food Additives: The Eat-Safe Guide.* Port Washington, NY: Ashley Books, 1980.

Karmel, Annabel. *Superfoods for Babies and Children.* New York: Atria Books, 2006.

Kent, Tami Lynn. *Mothering from Your Center: Tapping Your Body's Natural Energy for Pregnancy, Birth, and Parenting.* New York: Atria Books, 2013.

Kern, Deborah. *Everyday Wellness for Women.* Moulton, AL: Slaton Press, 1999.

La Leche League International. *The Womanly Art of Breastfeeding: Thirty-Fifth Anniversary Edition.* New York: NAL Dutton, 1991.

Lair, Cynthia. *Feeding the Whole Family: Recipes for Babies, Young Children, and Their Parents.* Seattle, WA: Sasquatch Books, 2008.

Lappe, Frances Moore. *Diet for a Small Planet: Twentieth Anniversary Edition.* New York: Ballantine, 1991.

Lipton, Bruce. *The Biology of Belief: Unleashing the Power of Consciousness, Matter and Miracles.* Carlsbad, CA: Hay House, 2008.

—. and Steve Bhaerman. *Spontaneous Evolution: Our Positive Future (and a Way to Get There From Here).* Carlsbad, CA: Hay House, 2009.

—. *The Honeymoon Effect: The Science of Creating Heaven on Earth.* Carlsbad, CA: Hay House, 2013.

MacWilliam, Lyle. *NutriSearch Comparative Guide to Nutritional Supplements.* Vernon, BC: Northern Dimensions, 2011.

—. *Comparative Guide to Children's Nutritionals.* Vernon, BC: Northern Dimensions, 2004.

McCann, Jennifer. *Vegan Lunch Box: 130 Amazing, Animal-Free Lunches Kids and Grown-Ups Will Love!* Philadelphia, PA: Da Capo Press, 2008.

Mindell, Earl. *Earl Mindell's Food as Medicine*. New York: Simon and Schuster, 1994.

—. *Vitamin Bible*. New York: Warner Books, 1992.

Morell, Sally Fallon and Thomas S. Cowan. *The Nourishing Traditions Book of Baby & Child Care*. Washington, D.C.: New Trends Publishing, 2013.

National Research Council. *Diet, Nutrition and Cancer*. Washington, DC: National Academy Press, 1982.

Newmark, Gretchen. "Eat That! Not!" *The Energy Times*, March/April 1994, pp. 40-44.

Nonken, Pamela P., and S. Roger Hirsch, M.D. *The Allergy Cookbook and Food-Buying Guide*. New York: Warner Books, 1982.

Northrup, Christiane, M.D., *Women's Bodies, Women's Wisdom*: *Creating Physical and Emotional Health and Healing*. New York: Bantam Books, 2010.

Northrup, Christiane M.D. with Kristina Tracy. *Beautiful Girl: Celebrating the Wonders of Your Body*. Carlsbad, CA: Hay House, Inc., 2013.

Ornish, Dean. *Dr. Dean Ornish's Program for Reversing Heart Disease*. New York: Random House, 1990.

Pert, Candace. *Molecules of Emotion: The Science Behind Mind-Body Medicine*. New York: Scribner, 1997.

Physicians Committee for Responsible Medicine. *Vegetarian Starter Kit*. Washington, DC, 2005.

Pollan, Michael. *In Defense of Food: An Eater's Manifesto*. New York: Penguin, 2008.

Pryor, Karen. *Nursing Your Baby*. New York: Pocket Books, 1991.

Rapaport, Howard G., M.D., and Shirley M. Linde. *The Complete Allergy Guide*. New York: Simon and Schuster, 1970.

Rapp, Doris J., M.D. *Allergies and the Hyperactive Child*. New York: Sovereign Books, 1979.

—. *Allergies and Your Family*. New York: Practical Allergy Research Foundation, 1990.

—. *Is This Your Child? Discovering and Treating Unrecognized Allergies in Children and Adults*. New York: William Morrow and Company, 1991.

Robertson, Laurel, Carol Flinders, and Brian Ruppenthal. *The New Laurel's Kitchen: A Handbook for Vegetarian Cookery and Nutrition*. Berkeley, CA: Ten Speed Press, 1986.

Rosas, Debbie, and Carlos Rosas. *The Nia Technique: The High-Powered Energizing Workout that Gives You a New Body and a New Life*. New York: Broadway Books, 2004.

Rosenberg, Marshall. *Nonviolent Communication: A Language of Life*. Encinitas, CA: PuddleDancer Press, 2003.

Rosenthal, Joshua. *Integrative Nutrition*. New York: Integrative Nutrition Publishing, 2007.

Roth, Geneen. *Women, Food and God: An Unexpected Path to Almost Everything*. New York: Scribner, 2010.

Roth, Ruby. *Vegan Is Love: Having Heart and Taking Action*. Berkeley, CA: North Atlantic Books, 2012.

Sanders, Tab, and Sheela Reddy. "Vegetarian Diets and Children." *American Journal of Clinical Nutrition* 59 (May 1994): pp. 1179-1182.

Sass, Lorna J. *Recipes from an Ecological Kitchen: Healthy Meals for You and the Planet*. New York: Morrow, 1992.

Silver, Tosha. *Outrageous Openness: Letting the Divine Take the Lead*. Alameda, CA: Urban Kali Productions, 2011.

Simkin, Penny, and April Bolding, Janelle Durham, Janet Whalley, and Ann Keppler. *Pregnancy, Childbirth, and the Newborn: The Complete Guide*. Minnetonka, MN: Meadowbrook Press, 2010.

Smith, Melanie M., and Fima Lifshitz, M.D. "Excess Fruit Juice Consumption as a Contributing Factor in Nonorganic Failure to Thrive." *Pediatrics* 93 (March 1994): pp. 438-43.

Surén, Pal et al. "Prenatal Folic Acid Supplementation Associated with Lower Risk of Autism." *Journal of the American Medical Association* 309(2013): 570-577.

Tate Firkaly, Susan. "Nutrition in Pregnancy." *Baby Talk*, May 1987, p. 24.

Tate, Susan. *Wellness Wisdom: 31 Ways to Nourish Your Mind, Body, & Spirit*. New York: iUniverse, Inc., 2011.

Thomas, Anna. *The Vegetarian Epicure*. New York: Vintage Books, 1972.

Thomas, Latham. *Mama Glow: A Guide to Your Fabulous Abundant Pregnancy*. Carlsbad, CA: Hay House, Inc., 2012.

Tolle, Eckhart. *Stillness Speaks*. Novato, CA: New World Library, 2003.

Toth, Robin. *Naturally It's Good . . . I Cooked It Myself!* White Hall, VA: Betterway Publications, 1982.

—. and Jacqueline Hostage. *Does Your Lunch Pack Punch?* White Hall, VA: Betterway Publications, 1983.

Vigdor-Hess, Wendy. *Sweetness Without Sugar: A Resource Guide for Delicious Dairy-, Egg- and Gluten-Free Treats Made with Healthy Sweeteners*. Afton, VA: SolThea Press, 2011.

Wasserman, Debra, and Reed Mangels, Ph.D., R.D. *Simply Vegan*. Baltimore, MD: Vegetarian Resource Group, 2006.

Weaver, Libby. *Accidentally Overweight: Solve Your Weight Loss Puzzle*. Auckland, New Zealand. Little Green Frog Publishing Ltd, 2010.

Weed, Susun S. *The Wise Woman Herbal for the Childbearing Years*. Woodstock, NY: Ash Tree, 1985.

Weil, Andrew. *Spontaneous Healing: How to Discover and Enhance Your Body's Natural Ability to Maintain and Heal Itself.* New York: Ballantine, 1995.

Weisenthal, Debra Blake. "Herbs for Pregnancy." *Vegetarian Times*, June 1994, pp. 86-87.

Wentz, Dave, Myron Wentz, Ph.D., and Donna K. Wallace. *The Healthy Home: Simple Truths to Protect Your Family from Hidden Household Dangers.* New York: Vanguard, 2011.

Williamson, Marianne. *A Course in Weight Loss.* Carlsbad, CA: Hay House, Inc., 2010.

Wolfe, Karen, and Deborah Kern. *Create the Body Your Soul Desires: The Friendship Solution to Weight, Energy and Sexuality.* Mission Viejo, CA: Healing Quest, 2003.

Wunderlich, Ray C. *Improving Your Diet.* St. Petersburg, FL: Johnny Reads, 1976.

—. *Nourishing Your Child: A Bioecological Approach.* New Canaan, CT: Keats Publishing, 1988.

Yarema, Thomas, M.D., Daniel Rhoda, and Chef Johnny Brannigan. *Eat-Taste-Heal: An Ayurvedic Guidebook and Cookbook for Modern Living.* Kapaa, HI: Five Elements Press, 2006.

Yntema, Sharon K., and Christine H. Beard. New *Vegetarian Baby.* Ithaca, NY: McBooks Press, 2000.

# About the Author

SUSAN TATE loves being a mother and a grandmother and treasures those titles above all others. A respected health educator for over forty years, she is widely recognized for being a wellness expert who inspires healthy choices from an empowering, loving, and compassionate perspective. That perspective was evident when she wrote the first edition of *Into the Mouths of Babes* in 1984. It was one of the first infant nutrition books ever published to offer guidance and recipes for feeding babies a healthy vegetarian diet. Susan is also the author of *Wellness Wisdom: 31 Ways to Nourish Your Mind, Body, & Spirit*; *AIDS & HIV Education: Effective Teaching Strategies*; and *Working Together to Prevent Sexual Assault*.

After moving to the Pacific Northwest in 2000, she founded Washington Wellness Associates. Prior to that time, Susan served as the director of health promotion and assistant professor in the School of Medicine at the University of Virginia for many years. She is a certified black belt Nia instructor who teaches internationally and delights in being known as a dancing grandmother. Her passion for her work is evident in her life's intent—to inspire individual, community, and global wellness. Susan lives in the Seattle area.

Washington Wellness Associates
www.wawellness.com

Into the Mouths of Babes
www.intothemouthsofbabes.com

# Index

Institute for the Psychology of Eating, 87

Iodine, 34, 51

Ipecac syrup, 189

Iron, 33-34, 51-52, 71, 73, 191

## J

Joy, the Sacred Nutrient, 55-56, 63

Juice:

added sugars, 74

diluting, 72, 74, 78

high intake, 74

## K

Kitchen layette:

preparation, 4

serving and storing 5

travel, 5

## L

Lacto-ovo vegetarian, 41

Lactose intolerance, 58, 79, 93, 98

La Leche League International (LLLI), 7, 67-68, 70, 72

Lipton, Bruce, 93-94

Love, in home-prepared foods, 2

Love, the Sacred Nutrient, 63-64

Low-fat, 39

Low glycemic, 25, 27-28, 33, 43-44, 84

Low-milk syndrome, 68

## M

Magnesium, 51

Mayo Clinic, 21, 98

Methemoglobinemia, 75

Microwave safety tips, 5, 105

Midwife, 20, 38, 67-69

Milk:

allergy vs. intolerance, 97-99

introducing baby to, 89, 97

Milk-free diet:

foods to avoid, 98-99

Minerals:

infants, 50-52

pregnant mothers, 30-35

Mood:

blood sugar levels, 25, 37

omega-3 fats, 30

Multiples:

weight gain in pregnancy, 20, 22

breastfeeding, 68

## N

National Eating Disorders Association, 86

National Foundation of Celiac Awareness, 101

Nausea, during pregnancy, 38

Nia, 22, 37, 87, 195, 207

Non-GMO, 14, 16, 29, 33, 59, 65, 71, 79, 102

Northrup, Christiane, MD, 35, 57, 86

Nourishing story, creating your, 24-26

Nourishment tips for pregnant moms, 38-39

Nutrients:

# Recipe Index